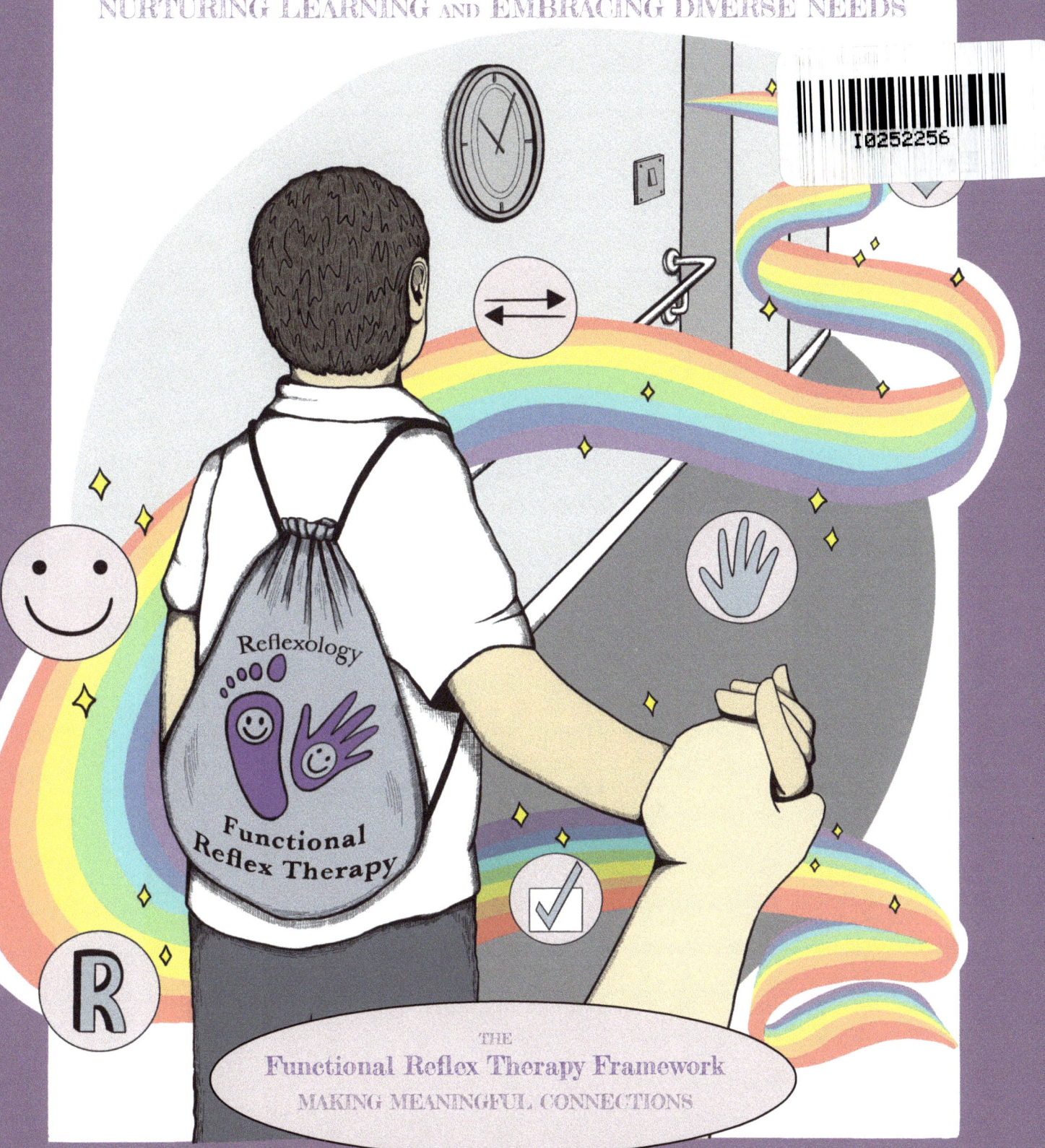

Copyright © 2023 by Lorraine Senior. All rights reserved.

This book or any portion thereof may not be reproduced or used in any manner whatsoever without the express written permission of the publisher except for the use of brief quotations in a book review.

Strenuous attempts have been made to credit all copyrighted materials used in this book. All such materials and trademarks, which are referenced in this book, are the full property of their respective copyright owners. Every effort has been made to obtain copyright permission for material quoted in this book. Any omissions will be rectified in future editions.

Cover image and illustrations by Catherine Taylor
Book design by: SWATT Books Ltd

Printed in the United Kingdom
First printing, 2023

ISBN: 978-1-7384466-0-5 (Paperback)
ISBN: 978-1-7384466-1-2 (eBook)

Lorraine Senior
Dunmow, Essex

www.functionalreflextherapy.co.uk

Contents

Acknowledgements	vii
Dedication	ix
Endorsements	xi
Disclaimer	xv
Author's Note	xvii
Prologue: Looking Back	xix
1 Welcome	**1**
Supporting the Educational Environment	1
My Aim for This Book	2
2 The FRT Framework	**5**
Supporting Complex and Diverse Needs	6
Why I Created the FRT Framework	7
3 How FRT Works	**9**
Simple and Uncomplicated	9
The FRT RECIPE for Success	10
The Delivery	11
The FRT Story Board: A Flexible Narrative	11
The FRT Toolkit	14
The FRT Logo	14
4 The Benefits of Reflexology on the Timetable	**17**
Being Accountable	18
Names, Labels, and Conditions	19
A Little Reminder	19
Becoming a Valued Member of the Multidisciplinary Team	20
5 A Little Bit of Science	**23**
The Impact of Anxiety and Stress	24
Perceiving a Threat	24
Signs of Stress	25
The Influence of Stress on the Nervous System	26
Gathering and Processing Information	27
'Happy' Chemicals	28
Studies and Research	30
6 Emotional Well-being, Consent, and Connection	**33**
Never Assume	33
The Process	33
How Do the Sessions Run?	35
Meaningful Communication	36

How Many Sessions?	39
Feedback	39
7 An Invitation to the Therapy Room	43
Presenting a Case Study	43
8 Meet George	45
The Process	46
Feedback from George	52
Gratitude and Learning	53
Links and Further Information	53
9 Meet Harry	55
The Process	56
Feedback from Harry	60
Gratitude and Learning	62
Links and Further Information	62
10 Meet Scott	63
The Process	64
Feedback from Scott	68
Gratitude and Learning	69
Links and Further Information	69
11 Meet Oliver	71
The Process	72
Building a Relationship and Lifting Self-esteem	73
Feedback from Oliver	75
Further Feedback from Oliver	76
Gratitude and Learning	78
Links and Further Information	78
12 Meet Harley	79
The Process	80
Feedback from Harley	85
Gratitude and Learning	86
Links and Further Information	86
13 Meet Cedric	87
The Process	88
Feedback from Cedric	92
Gratitude and Learning	93
Links and Further Information	93
14 Meet Kayleigh	95
The Process	96
Feedback from Kayleigh	100
Gratitude and Learning	101
Links and Further Information	101
15 Meet Dan	103
The Process	104
Feedback from Dan	107
Gratitude and Learning	109
Links and Further Information	109
16 Meet Suzzie	111
The Process	112

Feedback from Suzzie	115
Gratitude and Learning	116
Links and Further Information	116
17 Meet Fred	117
The Process	118
Feedback from Fred	123
Gratitude and Learning	124
Links and Further Information	124
18 Meet Sharmin	125
The Process	126
Feedback from Sharmin	131
Gratitude and Learning	132
Links and Further Information	132
19 Meet Charlie	133
The Process	134
A Few Words Shared from Charlie	135
Feedback from Charlie	139
Gratitude and Learning	140
20 When Headteachers and Reflexologists Meet	141
Harlow Fields School and College, Essex UK	141
Hayfield School, Merseyside UK	143
Reflexology at Transition2 in Derby UK	145
Youthreach, Kilkenny, Ireland	147
Endeavour Academy, Oxfordshire UK	149
Rowan Park Special School, Sefton UK	151
21 Final Words	153
Parting Gift	155
Where Do I Go from Here?	155
About the Author	157
Useful Resources	159
Bibliography	161

Acknowledgements

FIRST, I WOULD like to acknowledge the 200+ young people who have been invited to participate to receive reflexology at school, without whom the framework of Functional Reflex Therapy (FRT) would not have been developed. I would especially like to thank the inspiring young people you will meet in this book.

I offer thanks to staff, governors, and parents, past and present, of Harlow Fields School and College for welcoming me as part of the school community in the autumn term of 2011 and for their continued support and encouragement, giving me the space to develop reflexology with the FRT framework, the FRT Rainbow Workshops for parents and carers, the FRT Rainbow Relaxation Programme for the staff and the FRT Rainbow Self-Care well-being activity.

The Association of Reflexologists receives special thanks for its early recognition of the value of this therapeutic intervention, which really gave me the courage to move forward with it, and for honouring me with the first excellence award – Innovation in Reflexology 2016.

I would also like to acknowledge the growing number of qualified reflexologists who are members of the FRT network, and to thank you for your enthusiasm in using the framework to support your reflexology sessions.

I acknowledge, with grateful thanks, Widgit Symbols © Widgit Software Ltd 2002–2023 www.widgit.com for granting permission to use one of their symbols.

Finally, thanks to Catherine Taylor for her amazing skill in creating wonderful illustrations and for her patience in converting ideas from my mind (no mean feat!) and from photos into beautiful, unique visuals.

Dedication

TO MY WONDERFUL family, Hanna, Emily, and particularly my very tolerant husband, Martin, with much love and gratitude for putting up with my many notebooks, Post-it notes around the house, and constant ramblings often late into the night. (Although I'm not too sure he was always awake when he was resting his eyes!) For your great listening and supportive skills, Martin, and for nodding in all the right places, thank you. X

Endorsements

I FEEL VERY privileged to have three amazing professionals sharing their thoughts about this book, and words of support for my work, from different angles.

My first introduction to Lorraine's unique and powerful perspective on supportive reflexology using the FRT method of delivery and framework was back in 2013. We were both attending the Children's Complementary Network Conference. Lorraine's presentation taught me so much that continues to inform my own practice. She emphasised the importance of spending time in a structured way to enhance communication and reduce anxiety before the touch of reflexology. She showed a short video of a young man in the therapy room engaging with the FRT toolkit and enjoying time and meaningful communication to fully prepare him for his session. Ten years later and his smiling, relaxed face as he shared a real connection with Lorraine is still clearly in my mind. He felt valued, respected, reassured, and supported.

At the heart of this pioneering book are the stories of 12 remarkable young people who share the many benefits of receiving reflexology supported by the structured approach of the Functional Reflex Therapy framework within the school day. It feels a real privilege to be invited into the therapy room to meet these young people, each with challenging difficulties and diverse conditions, and to be part of their individual therapy experiences. The reader gets to know each young person and joins them in celebrating the many positive changes in their sense of well-being and ability to manage within the classroom.

The stories of the inspiring young people in this book show the value of time spent in awareness, not only before the session, but also during and afterwards. Within the structure of the approach there is time to gain consent to touch, time to choose the colour of a blanket and a comfortable position, for example. Time for the body to gather and process the touch of the slow, flowing, repetitive movements, and time to allow for a response. Time to listen and attend to verbal and non-verbal feedback and adjust for individual preferences. Time to reflect on the experience, share any worries or concerns, and maybe even enjoy a hug. And then time for the young person to return to the classroom feeling calmer, more confident, and in a better frame of mind for learning.

The power of the Functional Reflex Therapy method of delivery and framework lies in its structure and simplicity. While the efficacy of nurturing touch techniques cannot be underestimated, the emphasis is more on building meaningful connections through intention and mindful consideration of delivery. So often it is those shared experiences 'beyond touch' which encourage a positive change or shift within mood and behaviour that may be 'in the moment' or last much longer.

This book is essential reading for all reflexologists wishing to build on their existing skills by taking therapy into schools with a recognised, professional, and consistent approach. And it is of huge value to headteachers who are looking for ways to support the emotional well-being of their pupils. The book provides a wealth of evidence of the benefits of welcoming a qualified reflexologist into the team to deliver the therapy on the timetable during the school day.

I share Lorraine's firm belief that the therapeutic intervention of reflexology supported by the FRT Framework should be introduced to every school to help improve the well-being of young people during the school day and beyond.

Mary Atkinson, complementary therapist, author,
and co-founder of The Story Massage Programme
www.storymassage.co.uk

Lorraine provides us with the results of many years of experience and well-honed expertise.

This book is invaluable for any reflexologist or headteacher who wishes to work with, and support, children who have diverse additional needs and conditions. Lorraine clearly and concisely presents a well-documented and detailed plan of the care that she and her team have successfully offered to children with a range of ages and complex requirements.

The book introduces us to heart-warming accounts of treatment sessions, while Lorraine shares her thought processes and invites the reader to consider essential yet often missed details. My own years of working with babies and children leads me to concur with Lorraine's passion for sensitivity, patience, and respect for where each child is coming from.

I love the humour that she introduces as we, the readers, get to meet individual cases and Lorraine shares the minute details that made all the difference to the child.

This book serves as a guiding light, combining the power of reflexology with the principles of inclusivity to support children with diverse special needs. It deserves to be used as a foundational textbook in the care and development of children within a multidisciplinary approach, as the integration of reflexology in the support for all children has been long awaited. Everyone will win. The school has happier and calmer children while the children learn self-help techniques, or gain access to skilled one-to-one time with a trained FRT practitioner, and parents recognise that their child is gaining benefit by being happier and more relaxed and smiling more. As Lorraine herself says, she has learnt 'big time' from all those that she has supported throughout her extensive career by finding better ways to help children and schools achieve marvellous things together.

This is a ground-breaking book that opens doors to a whole world of introducing the therapeutic intervention of reflexology into the school day. In today's ever-changing world, the importance of inclusivity and support for children with diverse special needs cannot be overstated. Every child deserves the opportunity to thrive, grow, and reach their fullest potential. As we strive to create a more inclusive society, it is crucial that we provide holistic approaches to support their unique needs.

I have witnessed the potential of reflexology throughout the world and found that it is essential for children to be offered a safe and effective modality to support their well-being. These children may face unique challenges in their physical, emotional, and cognitive development and reflexology offers a valid way forward for them. This book maps it out for all to read.

I celebrate the fact that, with the help of Lorraine's FRT framework contained within this book, children will have the chance to express their inner world and schools will have the means to deeply help and support their children. The book emphasises the importance of individualisation and provides practical suggestions on adapting reflexology sessions to meet the unique requirements of each child. I know that by creating a nurturing and supportive environment, reflexology sessions can help children to develop a sense of self-awareness, improve their focus and attention span, and enhance their ability to regulate emotions. Lorraine is sharing her expertise with all for us to appreciate, and takes us along with her as she explores and provides deeply moving insights into her world, the educational establishments potential, and the individual's changes.

This book is as valid for schools as it is for reflexologists. The partnership between the two can achieve endless opportunities that can be monitored and measured. As you embark on your remarkable journey, may this book serve as a source of inspiration, knowledge, and practical tips. May it empower you to make a positive difference to the lives of all children through the transformative power of reflexology.

Sue Ricks, reflexologist, author, and founder
of The Gentle Touch of Reflexology
www.suericks.com

I am a firm believer that people come into our lives (personally or professionally) for a time (long or short) but definitely for a purpose. We may not always recognise this at first but, from the time Lorraine entered our school, I knew she would change our practice for the better!

What stood out at our first meeting was her smile, her calmness, and her overriding wish to use her reflexology skills to enhance the lives of our pupils.

Lorraine has been a teacher, understands schools, had worked with young people with learning difficulties, and she clearly 'got' our pupils. She didn't rush in with a 'this will fix it' attitude but took her time to have conversations with parents, staff, and pupils during which her calmness, warmth, and firm belief in reflexology were evident. Spending time with Lorraine lifted spirits.

With all her life experiences, Lorraine has the qualities to make her interactions with pupils, whether in schools in this country or abroad, so impactful. She has the ability to meet people where they are and this can be seen on every page – the time spent for small, but to us great, rewards is time very well spent!

This book will take you on a journey to revisit touch and to see how reflexology can be powerfully used as Functional Reflex Therapy. We know that touch has many benefits for both giver and recipient and can positively affect our communication with each other, our well-being, physical health, and emotional health.

It will show you how pupils who actively dislike touch and who wish to remain in control at all times can, with patience, time, and understanding, relinquish the control to allow themselves to benefit from two things we take for granted: communication and touch. You will see how Lorraine's training, research, and passion can change lives by giving our pupils the opportunity to discover choice making, communication, and, above all else, positive touch in their lives.

Functional Reflex Therapy is life changing and I am so pleased to have seen it in action with our very special pupils.

Kathleen Wall
Headteacher (2023)

Disclaimer

This book is not intended as a substitute for any medical advice and neither I nor the publisher can be held responsible for any loss or damage arising from any information contained in this book. Using the ideas shared within this book is the sole responsibility of the readers and at their discretion.

My apologies for any unintentional errors, which I will endeavour to correct in future editions.

Author's Note

ALL IDEAS AND experiences that have been brought together and shared in this publication are intended to help you, to inform you, and provoke your thinking. I accept that the work is my own personal subjective opinion, and, as such, it may not match the recollections or opinions of others.

Every effort has been made to provide up to date information that is as accurate as possible at the time of writing.

Although I refer to schools, colleges, and educational establishments, many strategies, discussion points, and suggestions are relevant and may be very suitable in many other areas of practice.

This is not recognised research, but I hope that the information presented here will act as a base to stimulate future research projects within this field.

The information within this book is not mine alone! It has been gleaned from my learning, my trials, from staff I have supported, from parents, tutors, and CPD courses from both my time in the world of education and the world of reflexology and, of course, most importantly, from the hundreds of wonderful young people I have supported.

Prologue: Looking Back

WHEN I CLOSE my eyes and give myself permission to allow memories to surface, to think of Little Highwood Hospital in the late 1970s, I picture the heavy green door looking scratched and in need of decoration. There's a small rectangular viewing window and, as I look through, I can clearly see little faces with beaming smiles appearing one after the other, their noses against the glass, as I waited for what seemed like ages for the door to be unlocked. They would often flatten their little hands on the window as if to say hello. I probably flattened my hand on that window too while I was waiting. It felt like a little connection and a lovely start to our morning together.

On entering the ward, I recall the bedheads were positioned against the wall along each side of the room, dormitory style. When I walked down the middle, I was always welcomed so enthusiastically by small hands, everyone wanting immediate attention. Giggles, noises, excitable sounds, a little speech, and a few pushes to try to get their hands into mine.

I had mixed feelings. Being wanted and feeling valued was great for me, but I recognised how desperate the young residents were for attention and nurturing touch and that brought me a tinge of sadness. I realised early on that staff (who were very few in number) simply didn't have the time to provide that.

I was 16 years old. Every Saturday morning around 6.30 a.m., I used to hop on my bike or – if I was lucky – I would persuade my lovely Dad to drive me several miles to the hospital, and what started as a six-month community activity towards the Duke of Edinburgh Silver Award continued for over two years!

The High Wood Workhouse and Little High Wood Hospital opened in Brentwood, Essex in the UK in 1904. At that time, it had five cottage-style wards, two schoolrooms and accommodated over 300 children with infectious diseases.

It was loaned to the War Office during the First World War and, after 1919, it continued as a place to treat children suffering with tuberculosis (TB) and rheumatic fever. Loaned again for support during the Second World War, it was later developed by the National Health Service as a place to continue its treatment for children with TB. As prevention methods improved and TB numbers declined, its use changed again. From the 1960s, the hospital accommodated 'mentally handicapped children' (a term used at that time), when I volunteered.

In those days, the children often had undiagnosed conditions. They were there because they were different. They were considered challenging, and some deemed ineducable. It's terrible to look back on this, but this was a time when those who were different were not accepted, often misunderstood, and families were embarrassed and had very little or no offers of support.

In my days at Little Highwood, I felt that my presence, time, kindness, and attention brought an additional quality into their young lives for a short period each weekend.

I usually sat on the floor, sang a lot, read stories, and sometimes I helped with feeding and dressing. Quite often my time seemed to be spent giving hugs and, although I didn't know much about the many benefits of positive and nurturing touch at that time, I knew I liked to receive it and so did many of the children. Many enjoyed hugs, sweeping movements along their arms and smiles often arrived when the tips of their fingers were gently squeezed and when their hair was stroked through or brushed.

Some watched from afar for a while and took their time to become familiar with seeing me regularly. I recall one young boy who watched our activities from a distance for many weeks. I would often see him bouncing on his bed with such energy. I remember the first time he came over and held out his hand, as if to say, 'I've watched long enough and now I'd like a go', and he allowed me to give it a little hello shake. In the following months he would frequently come over for a closer look, and sometimes stop long enough for a little squeeze on the ends of his fingers, then, he would dance off around the room, with a few happy delightful sounds, flapping and waving his favourite small piece of material.

We were, at times, on the receiving end of behaviours that were challenging, difficult for staff and very challenging to me as, to be honest, at that time I understood very little. One thing I learnt early on from that experience was that behaviours that were expressed were generally born out of sheer frustration. The young people often could not make themselves understood. Back then, we did not have many communication aids available to us, nor the knowledge and understanding of how to use them in a meaningful way. There was a lot of guesswork and assumptions made.

I stayed on at school into the sixth form for a couple of reasons; first, apart from art, I did not do very well with my exams. I needed to retake them and try again! And, second, I had no idea what I wanted to do. (I was instructed to work harder, which wasn't good for my confidence. A comment that has stayed with me most of my life.) Be careful with your words, people!

I needed to find my niche and some like-minded people. My best personal achievements and confidence were found on the hockey field and the netball court, particularly through the captain's duty to encourage others, or on the football pitch for the newly formed local girls' team, Warley Stars. I went to school longing for lunchtime and after-school sports clubs and joined in everything that was on offer. It was one of my sports teachers who suggested that PE College might be a way forward.

I applied for teacher training college and – to my amazement – was offered a place. Eventually, after many (and I do mean many) exam resits and a year out working at any job I could find, I went off to Dartford College of PE for four years. What an amazing learning curve it was, and I was very proud to graduate in 1986 with B.Ed Physical Education (PE) with (Hons).

In my final year, a new area of study became available, and I specialised in supporting children with motor impairment (as it was then titled). I went to teach PE in a mainstream secondary modern school in Rawtenstall in Lancashire for a couple of years, then undertook extra study at Manchester University, supporting children with Special Educational Needs. I moved into the special education environment in 1988, still with my PE hat on, to develop the movement and PE curriculum at Valley School in Bramhall, Stockport, and gradually developed my work to deliver classroom teaching in primary education. I remain so grateful to all the students and staff that have played such an important role in my learning and ongoing development.

Moves around the country led to new challenges and many exciting opportunities in a variety of special school environments. I feel privileged to have taught a wide range of ages in many education authorities, supporting young people with additional, complex, and diverse needs.

I always had an interest in complementary therapy and completed a basic course in aromatherapy massage in 1991. I delivered nurturing touch through simple massage movements in many of my own classrooms during my years of teaching, introducing relaxation sessions, and witnessing the many benefits that these sessions brought, not just to the person receiving the touch but also to the atmosphere within the classroom.

There's a saying that things happen for a reason, but often the reason is not easy to see or understand at the time. For me, it arrived with the early onset of osteoarthritis when I was in my early 40s; suffering pain and discomfort and restricted mobility, my hips would no longer allow me the freedom to run around the playground. I certainly did not see this coming! I could barely bend down in the classroom and if I did get down, I certainly struggled to get up. Nor could I continue with many of the sports I loved so much. For many years I was told by medical practitioners that there was nothing wrong. It was a difficult time and a bit of a downward spiral for all my plans and my mental health, as I had a young family who also had to cope with my reducing mobility and discomfort as it began to affect my day to day life. So, I took the decision to create another pathway.

I undertook more learning in the field of complementary therapy. I had received my first reflexology experience in 1995, loved it and bought *The Reflexology Handbook*, a wonderful book by Laura Norman, which had been sitting by my bed for 12 years! Now was the right time to put it to use, and I already had some dreams.

When I began training in reflexology I was presented with a short questionnaire about my expectations for the course and my aspirations in both the short and long term. All that before I had even started with any practical!

I still have that questionnaire and my answers (which bring a smile) dated 3 November 2007 and my response reads:

> *To step out of teaching and set up my mobile professional reflexology practice. I would like to explore the opportunity of working with people with special needs and those who have difficulty with their communication. Maybe bringing in some of my experience from the classroom but I have no idea how I can do this!*

So, along with the first of my two new hip replacements and after more than 20 years of teaching I did indeed step out, set up my private practice, and began to work on creating a professional package to highlight the value that reflexology could offer to support young people during the school day.

Alongside my general clients and mobile practice, I worked for a few years as a weekly reflexology volunteer with Mencap in Braintree, Essex, a charity that supports people of all ages who have a learning disability. I supported young people between eight and sixteen years of age at the Saturday playscheme.

It gave me the opportunity to build new relationships through reflexology and closely observe the responses. I used the sessions to combine movements and introduce and use specific methods of communication to help to give the young people a better understanding of what was happening before the touch, the importance of it, and the reasons why I was offering it to them. This was the time that I began to use social stories, communication symbols, and played around a little with the idea of the 'toolkit' to encourage those participating in the session to get more involved and put some of their favourite items into the bags too.

I am also extremely grateful to my beautiful Mum. As she struggled through her final years, tortured with vascular dementia, I was becoming confident enough about my skills and my understanding to deliver supportive hand reflexology. Mum loved a very gentle approach (not right for everyone but it was for her) and an approach that I had become familiar with through UK reflexologist and tutor Sue Ricks, with her Gentle Touch of Reflexology; it worked beautifully with my techniques and ideas. Importantly for me, I could observe Mum really closely and I recognised that the best responses came from increasing the repetition of the techniques. This was when I began to consider that there could be a protocol of delivery, which led me to reduce the number of changes of techniques and movements and increase the repetition of the delivery as I watched and listened carefully as I gave Mum time through repetition to feel each technique and become more comfortable as she became more familiar with the repetitive movements.

Mum would often ask, in her own way, for more of the movements that she really enjoyed. She seemed to recognise the towel as an indication it was our time together and what was going to happen. Maybe it was the towel itself or perhaps it was the colour (I don't know) but I always used the same colour and she seemed to like the texture and the soft feel of it. Sometimes she would help with the preparation and flatten it out, place her hands on it ready and she might smile. There were other occasions when she would just look straight at me, and if you are, sadly, familiar with complex neurological conditions, you may well have also experienced that stare, as the person you are supporting is trying so hard to make sense of the world around them. I'm pretty sure there were many occasions where she knew what she wanted to say but the words just wouldn't arrive.

I often just got on with organising and preparing and when I was ready, I would sit with my hands placed in an open position on the towel and invite her to participate, saying 'I am ready for your hands.' I remember I used to show the balm and place it to one side in view and, if she wanted it, she used to tap, tap, tap on the lid and tap, tap, tap some more if I took too long to follow her instruction.

Then, as the months passed, a time arrived during the later stages of her disease when I would just quietly and clearly explain, with very few words, each step that I was doing. We would then enjoy the touch and the time together. But I do know Mum took pleasure in receiving the touch and there was a calmness throughout her body. Occasionally an extra deep breath, a smile, and sometimes she used to lift my hand to her lips as if to give it a kiss. Although by this time I would often feel she didn't know who I was, I just found comfort in that Mum was deriving some enjoyment from the touch.

It wasn't all beautifully received, however, and sometimes situations changed quickly, like the flick of a switch. I learned, as you must when supporting your loved ones or clients with dementia, or any neurological challenge, not to take it personally. If possible, allow time, try again a few minutes later when you might be welcomed with smiles and love, and they will give their consent to receiving your touch. So, along with the work with the young people at Mencap, this all played an important part in my learning and in the development of the delivery that I use every day in school within my reflexology sessions.

I created a plan! I knocked on many school doors during my first few years. After much perseverance and, three years on, one of those doors did indeed open. I owe huge thanks and a debt of gratitude to the headteacher at Harlow Fields School and College in 2011. It is without doubt that I can say it was due to this opportunity, and the environment the school provided me with to develop my work over the following 12 years, that the FRT framework to support reflexology exists.

In 2013, I gave my first talk at a conference at Birmingham Children's Hospital to delegates from a variety of professions: therapists, teachers, medical practitioners. First, I couldn't believe my abstract had been selected! I was so nervous. It didn't help that I was the last presenter before lunch. Everything had already overrun and everyone was hungry, just to add to the pressure, but I did it! And the interest and encouragement I received was just what I needed to move forward; I was so thankful for that.

Full of enthusiasm, I introduced my first courses for reflexologists in 2014 in order to share my work and ideas, hopeful that they could see it supporting them and the development of their business.

The years flew by and, alongside my work in school and courses for reflexologists, there were some new FRT pathways to add to the training and some amazing experiences for me.

I wrote some articles for magazines and exhibited at events supporting special educational needs and disabilities in London and Norwich. Then I was invited to deliver a presentation at the International Council for Reflexologists Conference in Taiwan in 2017. I exhibited the many pathways of FRT at the Reflexology Conference UK in 2018, and a poster presentation at the ICR Conference in Alaska in 2019. As conferences and support went online, I was able to present to the Reflexology Association of America via Zoom in 2021. The latter had been due to be held in New Hampshire in 2020, but the world had other ideas!

As a result of the Covid-19 pandemic, Zoom has been, and continues to be, amazing for many, but I am pleased we are getting back together face to face and I am excited to welcome more reflexologists to join the training.

Together, we can work towards the FRT vision and ensure that every school in the world has a qualified reflexologist who uses the FRT framework to support young people who will benefit from our skills and expertise.

By the way, I achieved the Duke of Edinburgh Gold award in 1981 and thoroughly enjoyed a visit to the Throne Room at Buckingham Palace with the Duke of Edinburgh.

The Duke of Edinburgh scheme itself has changed a bit over the years but how apt that the programme now states that it is 'an opportunity to discover new interests and talents. A tool to develop essential skills for life and work'. When I look back at my career and timeline to date, I truly feel that the early experience at Little High Wood was the impetus for what I do today.

Chapter 1: Welcome

IN THIS BOOK, I invite you to our therapy room to experience the real-life challenges, achievements, and sheer joy as I share the many benefits of reflexology as it is successfully integrated into the school day, and how the structured professional package of the FRT framework and its RECIPE can support and underpin the work of the reflexology therapist.

I explore how you can use the framework to develop meaningful connections through touch and beyond, and how this supports the emotional well-being and wellness of young people with high levels of anxiety and diverse needs within the education environment.

This book is not merely a platform to share beautiful stories showing reflexology in action during the school day, although the stories do matter as they highlight its many benefits and are an integral part of the wholeness and vision for the book. It has been written to explain the efficacy, the worth, and effectiveness that the qualified reflexology therapist can bring to ease stress and calm the busyness of the mind and body 'in the moment'.

I show you why I believe so passionately that the therapeutic intervention of the nurturing touch of reflexology is so valuable that it should be available and accessible to all, in every school throughout the world.

Supporting the Educational Environment

The framework that supports reflexology which is shared in this book is flexible for all learning environments. I believe that wherever a young person participates in a learning situation is an educational environment, but, for the purpose of this book, I recognise the conventional learning environment is usually one of the following: a state funded school (in the UK this is free and provided by the government) or an independent school (often referred to as private). It generally supports children from primary school (at around five years old) through to secondary and college (around 19 years old), with both mainstream and/or special education support as the place where the majority of our young people spend most of their day.

I would like to think that the learning environment created would be a friendly one, where a person is given time and feels respected, safe, listened to, understood, and comfortable. These are generally agreed by all educators to be major factors to encourage the right frame of mind for learning to take place and for young people to thrive.

Our young people spend a high percentage of their early lives in the learning environment, so it would be right to create the best nurturing and supportive environment possible.

I think, like me, you would agree with Dorman *et al.* (2006), who suggest that 'Students learn better when they perceive the classroom environment more positively'.

However, while there are many amazing teachers and schools out there, they face some very big challenges in creating such a positive environment. This can make it very difficult for some of our young people to get by and to cope day to day, let alone be able to learn, to thrive, or to enjoy their school day. Of course, this makes it very difficult for our teachers too.

Challenges, to name just a few, include limited funding, appropriate and ongoing training, rising class sizes, and pressure to raise standards. Then there are challenges brought in from beyond the school gate, such as low self-esteem, being in pain or suffering discomfort, and medication that could unsettle a young person during the day or interrupt patterns of sleep. There may be difficulties where the young person is managing additional and complex health needs, profound and multiple learning difficulties, neurological difficulties, diverse differences and/or communication difficulties. Many of these may also co-exist or co-occur, all intensifying the workload and stress for the young people attending school and for the teacher and support staff.

However, this book has not been written to try to address the issues of the education system. It has been written to share my work and that of other reflexologists who use the many pathways of FRT to support their work. We all strive to help to make a little difference, supporting emotional well-being and wellness for some of our young people within the system as we currently find it.

We all have worries, frets, stress, and heightened levels of anxiety and we all manage them (or not) in different ways. They can be difficult at times for us to understand. We may find it hard to express the way we are feeling. It can be difficult to regulate and cope with our emotions and, at times, be hard to manage our behaviour.

We can all talk about what we want to happen in the future, and it is the responsibility of all of us to create a better system that will help reduce worries and frets and help young people better cope, manage, and thrive. But what about the young people that are currently working through the school system? The support is needed now!

My Aim for This Book

It is to explain my own unique perspective of reflexology. This book draws upon my personal experiences, my learnings, and the interpretations of others. It shows how you can provide supportive reflexology using the FRT method of delivery and framework.

This book is not designed to teach you about reflexology, and it is not designed to teach you everything I know. Instead, it shares the importance of the delivery of techniques, the intention of the work of the reflexologist, and building connections beyond the touch of reflexology. For this framework, it is about keeping it simple and making it meaningful.

I recognise and respect that every reflexologist comes with their own valid interpretation of techniques; there is no 'one size fits all', but I do ask for consideration of the method of delivery of the techniques (for good reason) and how they are linked together throughout the session when using this protocol.

Through the stories it shares, the many benefits of the FRT framework are revealed: its RECIPE (more on this later), the delivery of reflexology, and how bringing it together helps to create meaningful connections and works towards objectives beyond the touch.

There will be some brief outlines and examples of specific learning difficulties, conditions, and challenges that I have supported within my therapy room, the reasons I offer reflexology, the reasons the young people have been referred, the intention of my work and the expectations from me, from the person participating, from the team around this young person in school, and from the parent or carer.

While it is an important part of the role of a reflexology therapist to know as much background information as possible, which will include terms, labels, and conditions, it is not a dictionary of those things. I do not insist you use my language within your vocabulary – I am aware that the language in this book may not sit comfortably with everyone. All labels, names and terms are used with kindness and care, so please interchange any names and terms I use with ones you feel more comfortable with.

It is quite a minefield and sometimes confusing. I don't know how you feel but I personally feel there is an importance to giving a name to a condition. When it is used in a respectful way it can help the person receiving the name or diagnosis and it can help the people around that person. Then it becomes our responsibility to look at how we can best support them and what we may need to adapt.

The term used by Veronica Bidwell (2016) in her book, *The Parents' Guide to Specific Learning Difficulties*, describes my difficulties as she refers to a 'dizzying list of learning difficulties and conditions that seem to have emerged over the past decades'.

I think we all mean well but may not always choose or use the right wording or name. It is important to share our thoughts, be respectful, and keep discussions kind.

This book has been written primarily for reflexologists and highlights the value of being a qualified reflexologist and a valued member of the multi-disciplinary team in a school. In it, I share ideas you may consider useful to help you to feel more confident in allowing your reflexology to be accessible to all.

I introduce you to ideas that may help you to introduce your professional self and your reflexology business to headteachers and principals and to explain the many benefits of your reflexology therapy and the value you can offer within the school system. I also give you further information about training opportunities with FRT for you to decide if it can support you and the pathway along which you might like to take your reflexology business.

I appreciate that this book may also resonate with headteachers and staff, and I value giving you the opportunity to see and hear about the many benefits that are available through reflexology therapy. I encourage you to consider reflexology therapy in your school, where the reflexologist supports their work through the FRT framework.

I also share additional pathways of support that can be offered by the reflexologist through FRT, not just for the learners during the school day but also for staff and for parents and carers.

Chapter 2: The FRT Framework

I BEGIN THIS chapter by acknowledging that I recognise there are already reflexologists doing great work supporting young people in both the mainstream and the special education environments. But as great and as valuable as this work is, if you are working independently, it is likely that very few people know about your work outside the local community. Together we can change this.

When the word reflexology is used, I wonder what it means to you. I envisage a huge 'umbrella' of amazingness.

Reflexology has many different approaches, methods, and techniques. It is delivered in a multitude of ways to support numerous issues, difficulties, and conditions. It can be complicated and sometimes confusing to try to explain it to others, even for us as reflexologists.

But one thing, which is central to the 'hugeness' of the non-invasive caring and nurturing touch of reflexology, I think we can all agree on is how it affects the way people feel and how it can support well-being.

My reason for creating a professional package and giving it a name is to provide a clear intention and structure of reflexology specific for schools, enabling reflexologists to work in a similar way. It does not take away our individual skills and expertise, but it means there is a recognised protocol which lifts our professional standing as qualified reflexologists.

This framework, while supporting reflexology, does not detract from opportunities to be adaptable and flexible in order to meet diverse needs, but it brings clarity and consistency to the role of the reflexology therapist within the school environment. The aim is to have the value of the professional reflexologist recognised and encourage education authorities and headteachers to search for reflexology therapists to support the young people in their school.

I wanted to give the process a title, using words that would be meaningful for schools and that would begin to draw attention to the intervention under the huge umbrella of reflexology. 'Functional Reflex Therapy' was the result:

Functional because it has a structure, a purpose, and an intention.

Reflex because it relates to how the body receives messages through the stimulus of positive touch.

Therapy because it relates to activities undertaken to encourage a response or change throughout the body.

As the title of the book suggests, the work of a reflexologist in a school can bring meaningful connections in so many ways. The nurturing touch is supportive and should be accessible by anyone who is finding it difficult to regulate their emotions and cope during the school day. The framework, which highlights the touch and beyond, encourages the therapist to consider what methods may be used to support the touch of reflexology.

Supporting Complex and Diverse Needs

The idea for the framework developed as I delivered weekly reflexology therapy sessions with Mencap, supporting young people with learning disabilities. I had the opportunity to carry out several small studies (unpublished) between 2010 and 2012 in which I set out to explore the effects of relaxation reflexology techniques.

My young clients reminded me how important it was that I helped them to understand what was going to be happening in advance, so that they had time to prepare. It made me carefully question and consider my methods of communication so that it was appropriate and meaningful for each person. It reminded me how I needed to allow sufficient time for each person to prepare and to gather and respond to the information I was presenting them with.

Just as I had done with my lovely Mum, I watched, listened to, and observed carefully each step of the therapy session. I received feedback from the young people by observing how calm and relaxed they became, how much they began to enjoy the sessions, along with the positive responses from staff.

Generally, everyone returned to take part in the group activities in a calm state. Some seemed quite tired and took a little time out and some smiled, not really being able to share how they were feeling, but staff understood it to mean they had enjoyed the session and felt good. I use the word 'generally', because we can never truly say how the body might respond and there were occasions of heightened liveliness, sometimes a very quiet withdrawal or a little sadness with a release of emotions. It may have been an expression of how they were feeling at that moment in time, it may have been something they were thinking about that had happened perhaps earlier in the day or at another time, or what may have poured out of the body as they were allowed to be themselves.

Through this work, I began to think about the session before the touch, then during the touch and what worked well, and then how I finished it. It became clear that there were some important points that made this successful.

Why I Created the FRT Framework

A number of schools benefit from a combination of specialist therapy support, including occupational therapy, physiotherapy, speech and language therapy, play, art, and music therapy, and talking therapy, to name a few. All of these therapists work alongside teachers, and are using similar protocols across their professions, so the school knows what it is buying into and the intention of the service.

Currently, there are not many schools in which reflexology therapy is used, and few advertising for a reflexology therapist, which means they are missing a valuable addition to their multi-disciplinary team to help them access the needs of some of their pupils.

By providing the FRT framework to support reflexology, my aim is to help reflexologists to develop their business within this environment and make it easier for headteachers to talk and share information with other headteachers about the value of the therapy within school.

FRT has its own specific *modus operandi* with its supportive framework and method of delivery of the reflexology, which is explained in detail in the coming chapters.

Chapter 3: How FRT Works

Now you know why I created it; I will continue in this chapter to explore the different parts of the process to show how it adds value and the ease with which it can be implemented during the school day. There are three vital points the reflexologist needs to address for its success.

1. Your preparation and communication, how you help the young person you are inviting for reflexology to feel comfortable and to understand what is happening, and how you encourage them to get involved and engage.

2. The method of the delivery of the reflexology techniques is very important. Consider how the body processes the communication of your touch. My strapline makes it easy to remember:

    More of less = more
    - more repetition of movements
    - less changes of techniques
    - = more response

3. Time underpins the whole process. Time to process information, time to prepare, time to feel the movements, time to respond, time to finish and prepare for the next activity.

Increasing the repetitions of each movement and reducing the changes of techniques allows the body time to feel and process the information communicated by the reflexologist through the modality of touch, resulting in a more positive response.

Simple and Uncomplicated

Two essential words I use when talking about the FRT protocol for reflexology in schools is that when you keep the approach *simple* and *uncomplicated* the rewards are amazing! When I question the efficacy, there are always positives to reflect upon, which are also recognised by teachers, support staff, and parents.

The FRT RECIPE for Success

Anyone else love a mnemonic? I hope it will not only bring a smile but help as an important reminder of what you need to consider: it is so much more than 'just' the touch of your reflexology.

You will see the icons from the R E C I P E throughout the stories. I wonder what points you will consider to be important, not just in my book with my examples, but when you prepare and plan your own sessions.

Following a recipe can, of course, refer to following a list or set of instructions and this brings out great discussion during training. The ingredients of the FRT R E C I P E are respect, empathy, communication, intention, preparation, and efficacy. Blend these ingredients to work for you and the person you are supporting, just as you will be doing with the techniques you use to create a therapy session that can best meet individual needs.

Take a little time to carefully consider each of these terms. Let me start you off. I look forward to our discussion.

 Respect: Giving respect, showing there is a value to the young people's feelings and wishes. Listen and act on their preferences. Thoughtfulness and consideration.

 Empathy: An understanding about another person, an awareness of their feelings, but, it's not your situation so think carefully about how you work with this.

 Communication: Sharing/giving information, but beware, it needs to be meaningful, and communication is both giving and receiving. Be an effective communicator.

 Intention: Ask yourself what your plan of support is and the aim or purpose of this session.

 Preparation: Getting yourself ready and helping the young person to get ready and to know what is happening with meaningful methods of communication.

 Efficacy: Be reflective and aware throughout and ask yourself how effective the session has been, and what value it has offered.

The Delivery

The professional reflexologist can use the basic FRT relaxation techniques and routine as a standalone therapy. However, it is more usual for it to be used as an additional support alongside more advanced and skilful specific reflexology techniques that the therapist considers beneficial to, and appropriate for, the young person they are supporting.

Using the FRT framework means every therapist is encouraged to start and finish using the protocol, giving clear information to the person taking part in the session that there is a beginning and an end. Therapists are encouraged to use the same linking effleurage movement between each technique and use increased repetition to each movement they give.

Linking the reflexology techniques with a calming movement that sends a 'slowdown' message throughout the body, we provide a combination of tactile information for the different receptors that are found within different parts of the skin. Signals are received by the mechanoreceptors, which are either slow in responding in the non-glabrous (hairy skin) or faster to respond in the glabrous (non-hairy skin), a combination that is important in the delivery of this method.

The FRT Story Board: A Flexible Narrative

When considering the whole therapy session we offer as reflexologists, it is not only the therapeutic touch that brings value, but also, undoubtedly:

- » the respect, kindness, and intention of our support, and the relationship we develop with our young clients as we get to know them;
- » it's not just working with them, but it is the real 'getting to know them' that has a significant impact on the success of the session;
- » how we prepare ourselves and how we prepare the person coming for the therapy;
- » how we support them throughout the session with appropriate communication that is meaningful for them and how we help them to prepare for the finish and their return to class;
- » how we adapt our techniques and create something that is right for them.

Of course, I know some readers will be questioning how much of the success is attributed to the framework and how much to the touch of reflexology. This is about reflexology with a framework to provide support during the school day. My opinion of this, to play 'devil's advocate', is that it does not matter how much success is due to the supportive framework and how much is due to the supportive reflexology. It is a combination, and I look forward to future discussions on this subject. In the meantime, enjoy following the the visual story and perhaps consider how you can adapt and integrate some of these ideas into your practice.

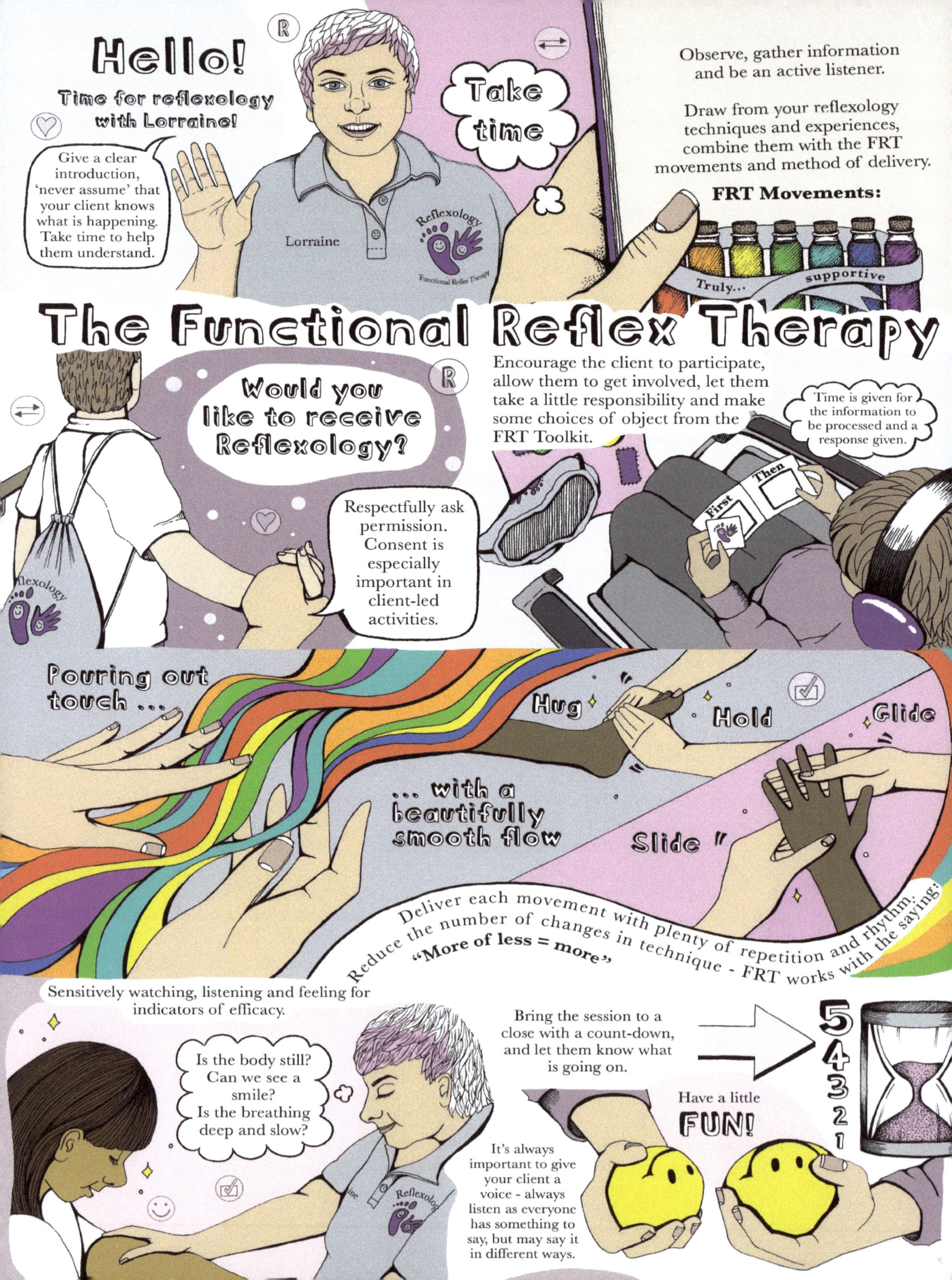

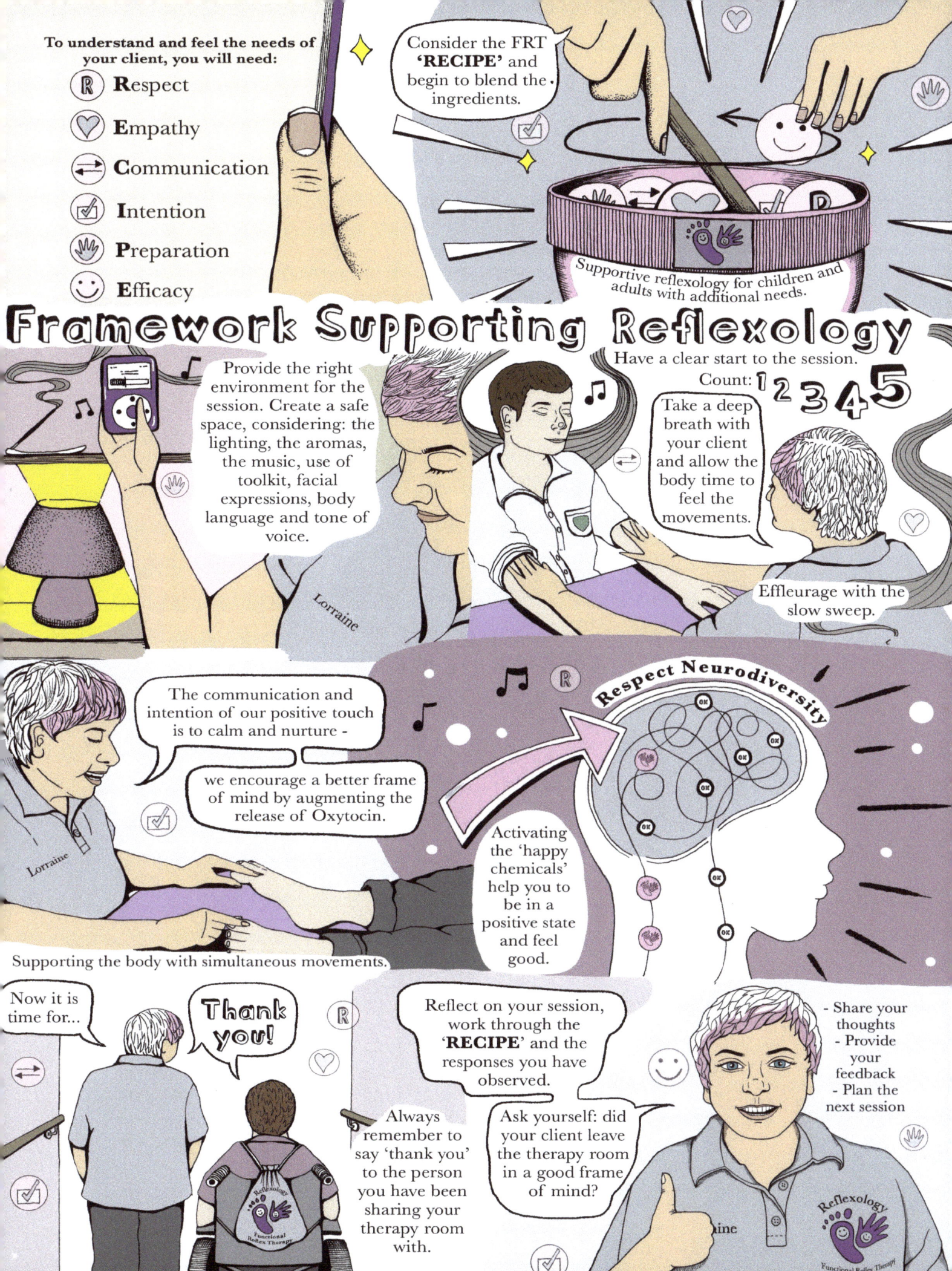

The FRT Toolkit

Sometimes, simple adaptations and additions encourage involvement, bring fun, help with communication, and may ease anxiety. The FRT toolkit is one such small addition with powerful supportive results, often for communication and preparation. (Remember the RECIPE.) The use of the toolkit is dependent on it being meaningful, but meaningful could entail fun and enjoyment and getting involved in the session from the classroom, which should not be underestimated. So, it is not always used but for some it is absolutely the right start to the session. It communicates that it is time for reflexology, a valuable object of reference. There is more about that in the stories when you meet the young people, where it can be really helpful for transitioning from one activity, or one area of the school, to another.

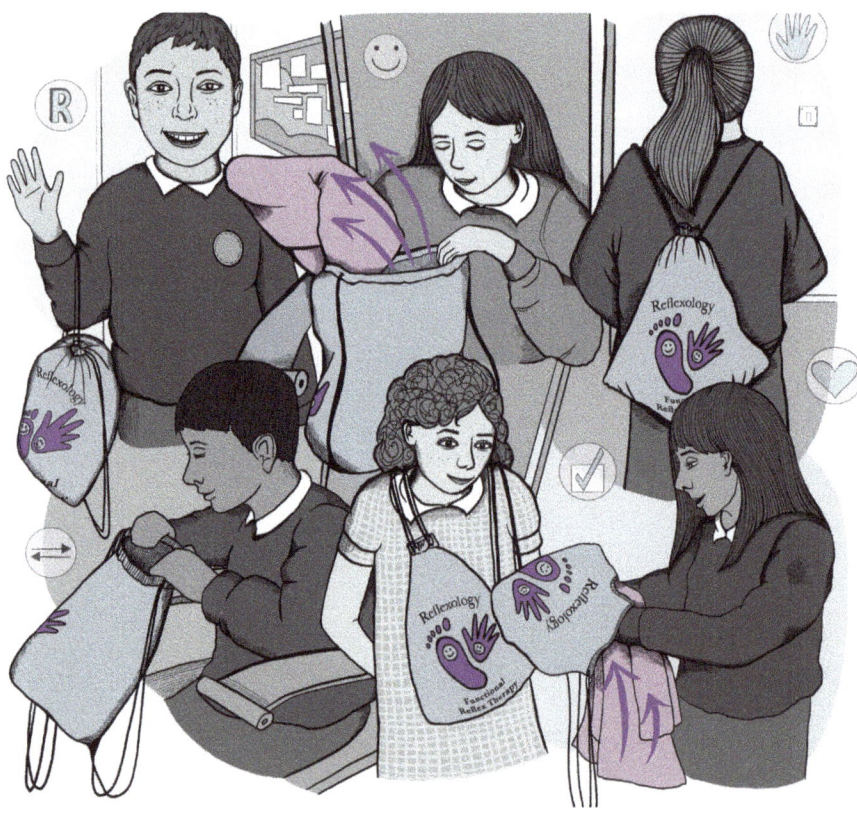

Preparation

Getting involved

Communication

Taking responsibility

Raising self-esteem

Being helpful

Giving a little control

The FRT Logo

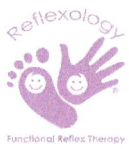 It's all about communication, it shows the foot and the hand, which are the areas I work with. We use the smiley face a lot in school, and I popped it into 'kind of' speech marks, again to represent communication. It's often interesting, as I walk along the corridor, to notice that many are drawn to the logo on my polo shirt,

sometimes stopping to give it a little prod as if to say I remember coming along, sometimes I get a little hug! Smiley faces can be used in many ways, and for my lovely Mum with her dementia, this was one of the things she loved looking at, especially on the squeezy balls!

Let me give you an example of how this works in practice. When Amanda, an FRT reflexologist, wanted to reduce her hours working in a school, she asked the FRT network if there was a therapist that would like some of those hours. When Seema stepped in and used …

- » the same structured start and finish to the session (there is more about that in the stories);
- » not always the same techniques but always a similar method of delivery, repetition, and the same linking movement;
- » the same intention and purpose for the sessions;
- » the same FRT polo shirt;
- » the same FRT toolkit;
- » the same logo;
- » similar recording and feedback …

it continued successfully. It is my understanding that Amanda and Seema never met face-to-face, but the school thought they knew each other, as they had such a similar successful approach. Of course, the children did notice it was a different person, but the approach stayed familiar, continued well, and the transition was smooth. Well done to both reflexologists! Well done to the FRT framework!

Chapter 4: The Benefits of Reflexology on the Timetable

THE REFLEXOLOGY THERAPY room and its positive touch, like many therapies, offers time and a safe, reassuring, calm, and comforting environment.

Our touch is often offered without any spoken words. Sometimes, in my therapy room, it is with photographs and gestures. It might be led by examples to follow, e.g., just sitting down and pointing, I have even removed my shoes and socks as we work together with appropriate communicative methods. It is always non-judgemental, with very few demands.

The therapy we can offer during the school day is uncomplicated, simple in its delivery, a calming sensory experience, and a supportive form of communication.

The benefits for young people receiving reflexology may include:

- releasing tension, creating relaxation and calm;
- giving the opportunity to express feelings;
- supporting emotional well-being;
- raising awareness of one's own body, proprioception;
- helping them to manage their own stress and anxiety;
- increasing their self-esteem;
- allowing them to feel in control of the activity and encouraged to give or not to give consent;
- managing better during the school day, as it may help with focus and concentration;
- taking time away from the busyness of the classroom;
- giving the opportunity to establish a new relationship;
- identifying if the experience is something they would like as part of their lifestyle outside of the school environment;
- learning some transferable self-care, supportive reflexology techniques;
- giving them the opportunity and time to enjoy the sensory experience and to feel good.

You will read about the importance of communication in all the stories, as well as the importance of creating meaningful connections.

The benefits for the school may include:

- having a more content young person, with lower tension, reduced levels of stress, increased concentration, and being in a better frame of mind for learning;
- supporting general well-being and perhaps reducing absenteeism;
- helping and improving the home–school link, as parents and carers can also be guided by the reflexologist to use supportive FRT relaxation in their own homes;
- using the therapy sessions to support individual learning targets, some of which you will read about in the stories. This may include the ability to make choices, developing language skills, following instructions, giving consent, taking responsibility, and so on;
- innovative therapeutic intervention support from a qualified reflexologist can lift a school's profile. This can be shared and discussed easily using the Functional Reflex Therapy framework protocol.

The purpose and primary objective are to ease the busyness of a young person's mind, to foster a more settled being, and promote a calmness that may help with self-regulation and self-management during the school day.

Being Accountable

To be successful, we need to be accountable! This is essential and necessitates taking different forms and pathways, as you will need to be able to share the value of reflexology being on the timetable.

The reflexologist will be accountable to:

- yourself, the ethos of your association/organisation, and your insurance company;
- the young people you are supporting;
- the teachers and staff;
- the school and governors;
- parents and carers;
- Ofsted (Office for Standards in Education) in the UK or similar institutions in other countries of the world.

Hence, it is essential that the reflexologist has guidelines in place as part of school documentation for reflexology supported by the Functional Reflex Therapy framework (support, templates and information are all available to FRT members to help with preparation of these important documents).

Names, Labels, and Conditions

A question I am often asked is 'Do I need to be a specialist to understand the issues and complexities of conditions, differences, disorders, disabilities and difficulties, names, terms, and labels?' It can feel very daunting.

As reflexologists we are very aware that each client who comes into our therapy room is unique, and we try to organise ourselves to be ready and as flexible as possible to support in whichever way we feel our client may need.

This book is not a dictionary of definitions; it does not focus on descriptions of conditions, names, labels, or terms, but they are important for me to mention and those used will undoubtedly carry varying degrees of significance and resonate with us all differently. For example, I know some people reading this will refer to 'young people who have autism', while others will refer to 'a young person who is autistic'. I recognise this diversity and ask you, the reader, to reframe and allow yourself to use vocabulary that works for you.

I do believe we should think of these terms as opening doors for us to access supportive practices, therapies, and/or education. There are many terms, labels, and conditions and they may have a second diagnosis and other medical conditions, which are usually referred to as co-occurring or co-existing.

Collecting background information and learning as much about a young person as possible is very important and necessary for the reflexologist to gain a comprehensive understanding, which will be crucial to the success and effectiveness of their approach. However, the main purpose and intention of the reflexology session during the school day, regardless of all the background information, conditions, and labels, will always remain consistent when using this framework.

A Little Reminder

The benefit of receiving reflexology during the school day, supported with the FRT framework, is that it helps these young people with the management of their anxieties, aiding calmness and relaxation, and encourages them to return to the classroom in a better frame of mind.

A question I am often asked is: Can you work with anyone? You may consider there are contra-indications for your therapy; ultimately, this will be your decision, but do ask yourself what is the intention of your session and what is stopping you from offering the support.

Remember that in all your sessions, touch and time can be flexible and adapted. Young people who are receiving medication(s) can successfully take part in the reflexology sessions with the main aim being to allow them to become calm and relaxed and bring about as much balance as possible. It should not be underestimated that the medications prescribed, which may sometimes be taken in high dosages, may be the cause of the stress and anxiety within the body and have an impact on the immune system and emotions. Ultimately, the value of easing the stress and calming the body and mind with kindness, care, time, and touch, establishing a meaningful connection, must not be underestimated.

In our capacity as reflexologists, it is not our responsibility to try to address the label of a condition that has been given to the young person we are working with. But, as I have already mentioned, it is imperative to learn about each person and their challenges, difficulties, and disorders in order to tailor, adapt, and blend the ingredients of the FRT R E C I P E and the delivery of our therapy to best support their well-being and help them to better manage situations throughout the school day.

Reflexologists – it is important to do your homework and preparation. Collaborate with parents and staff and develop your awareness and understanding about medical conditions, labels, and diagnoses. This is all vital background information and may have an effect on how you adapt your room or your approach, both in and out of the therapy room throughout the framework, but do not lose sight of the intention of the session and why you are delivering it during the school day.

Becoming a Valued Member of the Multidisciplinary Team

Many of the young people you will be supporting will have complex medical and educational needs, and because of this they may have a large team of professionals around them providing support and services. It is important to co-ordinate and communicate with this team so that the best support is provided and the young person is not overwhelmed with too much support.

Over the years, many parents, carers, and families have mentioned the energy needed to constantly repeat information about their child, which is so challenging. I personally remember this issue when caring for my parents and seeing numerous consultants, doctors, and therapists and this was over a relatively short period of time. This was helpful, along with advice from reflexologists during the early development of FRT, when designing the questionnaire specifically for parents and carers, which is additional to the consent form.

I have also designed a similar yet different questionnaire for teachers and support staff. This brings information and insights from both the home and school environments, raising awareness of different perspectives, and I can follow up and ask questions if I need further information, advice, or clarification.

Although it is not obligatory to return the questionnaires, as is the case for the consent forms, to date all the questionnaires have come back and have been very helpful. It is always interesting to receive information from home and school and always important to be respectful of both points of view, which sometimes can be very different.

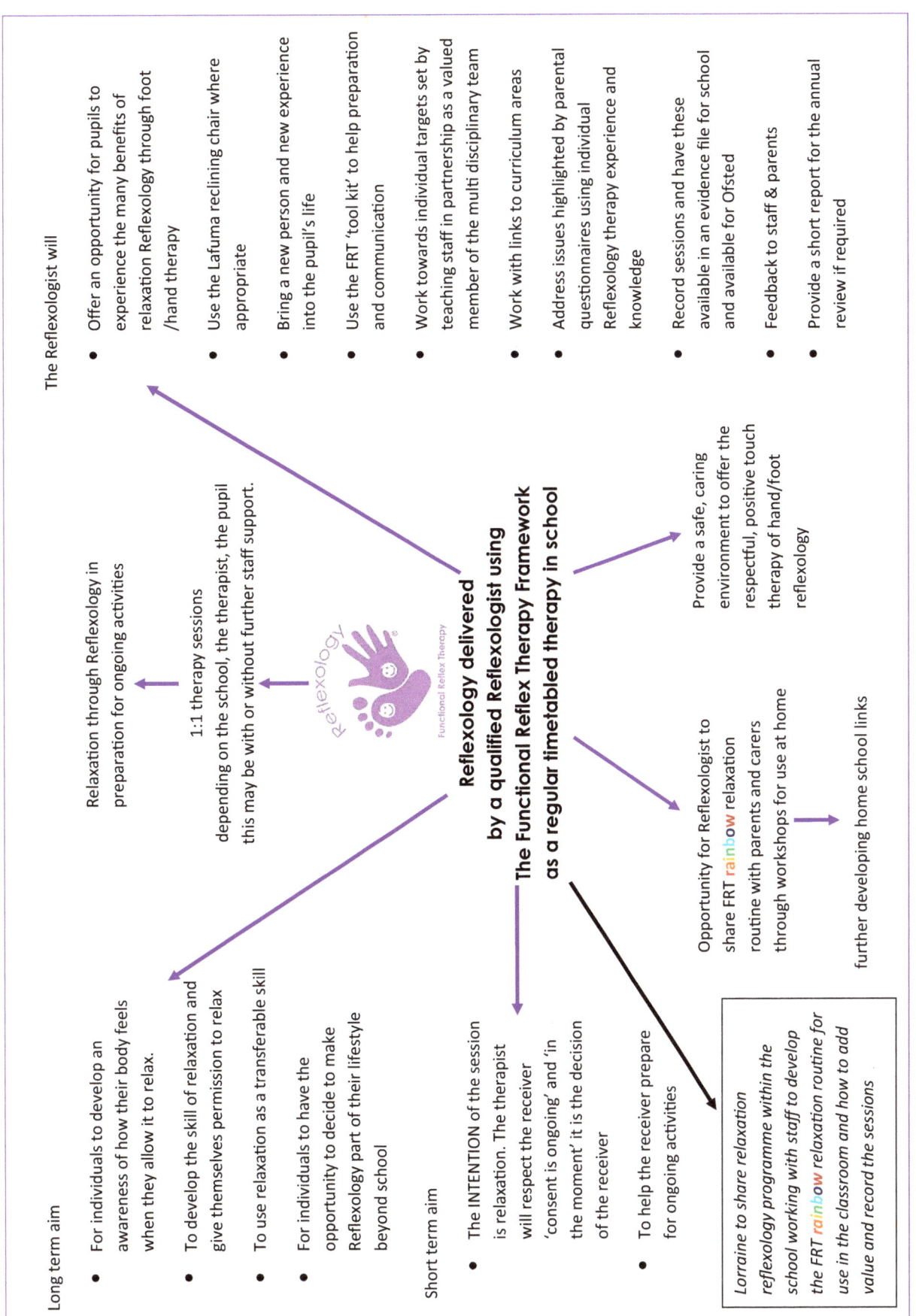

Reflexology delivered by a qualified Reflexologist using The Functional Reflex Therapy Framework as a regular timetabled therapy in school

Long term aim

- For individuals to develop an awareness of how their body feels when they allow it to relax.
- To develop the skill of relaxation and give themselves permission to relax
- To use relaxation as a transferable skill
- For individuals to have the opportunity to decide to make Reflexology part of their lifestyle beyond school

Short term aim

- The INTENTION of the session is relaxation. The therapist will respect the receiver 'consent is ongoing' and 'in the moment' it is the decision of the receiver
- To help the receiver prepare for ongoing activities

Lorraine to share relaxation reflexology programme within the school working with staff to develop the FRT rainbow relaxation routine for use in the classroom and how to add value and record the sessions

Relaxation through Reflexology in preparation for ongoing activities

1:1 therapy sessions depending on the school, the therapist, the pupil this may be with or without further staff support.

The Reflexologist will

- Offer an opportunity for pupils to experience the many benefits of relaxation Reflexology through foot /hand therapy
- Use the Lafuma reclining chair where appropriate
- Bring a new person and new experience into the pupil's life
- Use the FRT 'tool kit' to help preparation and communication
- Work towards individual targets set by teaching staff in partnership as a valued member of the multi disciplinary team
- Work with links to curriculum areas
- Address issues highlighted by parental questionnaires using individual Reflexology therapy experience and knowledge
- Record sessions and have these available in an evidence file for school and available for Ofsted
- Feedback to staff & parents
- Provide a short report for the annual review if required

Provide a safe, caring environment to offer the respectful, positive touch therapy of hand/foot reflexology

Opportunity for Reflexologist to share FRT rainbow relaxation routine with parents and carers through workshops for use at home

→ further developing home school links

Short-term and long-term goals are important to highlight the value and many benefits of having a reflexologist as part of the school team and sharing information easily. Consider creating something similar to the example shown in the diagram on the previous page as a valuable addition for your school development plan. This is a helpful resource to refer to for staff, governors, and perhaps visitors.

Chapter 5: A Little Bit of Science

REFLEXOLOGISTS USING THE concept of the FRT framework will predominantly support young people who have additional, complex, and diverse needs. As I mentioned in the previous chapter, these young people may be autistic, have profound and multiple learning difficulties, be diagnosed with a learning or intellectual disability, and have language, communication, and/or information processing difficulties. All the young people (whatever labels they may or may not come with) are displaying anxiety, worries, and frets and are in a difficult frame of mind to cope during the school day. Or perhaps a better way to phrase this is that they have difficulty coping with the world around them in a way that society expects and accepts, both inside and outside the world of education. It may be a good place here to justify the choice of my wording in my title. I have specifically used the wording 'diverse needs' as my intent to acknowledge and embrace inclusivity as we recognise that any point any young person with any level of ability, with any label, with any condition could experience challenges which will have an impact on how they manage during the school day and reflexologists have a valuable method of support and can provide various FRT pathways of assistance.

However, understanding some of the conditions and how the body gathers and processes information is paramount and the reason there is a unique delivery method and approach within the framework of FRT.

We know the brain is a very complex organ, controlling every process that regulates the body. There are areas, parts, lobes, glands, masses, sections, groups, tracts, capsules, bundles, bands, fissures, ganglia, and nuclei, which all intricately work together, but they do have some more general specific roles and responsibilities.

There are many wonderful tutors and textbooks that can share the workings of the brain. I do not possess expertise in this area, and I am not going to attempt to detail it in my book, but it is worth mentioning a little about the brain as it does underpin my work with reflexology and FRT and its framework, so it is important to dip in. I hope it will provide an opportunity for further learning and encourage much discussion.

Lorraine Senior

The Impact of Anxiety and Stress

We talk about anxiety and stress a lot in society. But what actually is it? MIND – a mental health charity originally founded in 1946 when it was named the National Association for Mental Health (NAMH) – states that 'Anxiety is what we feel when we are worried, tense or afraid – particularly about things that are about to happen, or which we think could happen in the future' (Mind.org.uk).

Most of us have times when we feel anxious, and we all deal with these feelings differently. If we recognise it quickly enough, it is likely that we can put strategies in place to help us cope with these feelings. However, we may not even realise that our actions or feelings may be placed under the term anxiety.

Dr Luke Beardon, author of *Avoiding Anxiety in Autistic Children: A Guide for Autistic Wellbeing*, asks the question 'How do autistic children experience anxiety?'

It is a fascinating and mind-opening read and he suggests that 'you make time to try to appreciate if you do not suffer from anxiety in your everyday life that will be very difficult to try to empathise with a person who does'. He goes on to say that 'it is vital to try to understand on some level how someone else might be feeling so that you can better support them'.

Of course, anxiety doesn't exclusively affect people who are autistic; it affects many young people and may have an impact on how they manage and cope with demands and activities throughout the school day.

Beardon goes on to state that 'If a child is exposed to stress on an ongoing basis for prolonged periods of time, then the risk of developing complex anxiety increases'. He suggests we should take the term anxiety extremely seriously because 'the more a child is exposed to anxiety = the greater risk of long-term complex mental health problems', statements with which I think we can all agree.

Perceiving a Threat

Whenever anyone perceives that there is a challenge or a threat in a physical or emotional way, the body initiates, and triggers, a stress response. This reaction may have an effect and impact areas of the brain that are responsible for managing and regulating emotions and help with organisation, which can cause many of the issues and stress responses we observe or refer to as causing challenges during the school day. These stress responses can be defined as:

Fight – the fight response may be aggressive behaviour, trying to fight as a response, maybe shouting at someone or something and hitting out.

Flight – the flight response is to run away to avoid the demand, the challenge, whatever is perceived as the threat.

Freeze – we don't often talk about the freeze response, but it happens if the fight or the flight are not seen as the right option. What some people may do is completely stop and hope they do not have to deal with the request or the situation.

Fawn – the fawn response is when young people do not focus on their own health and well-being needs and what they want, in order to please others.

This is a complex area that will have an impact on how some of our young people cope or manage during the school day. With all this in mind, think about the intention the reflexologist brings to the session and the support they may be able to offer, working alongside other members of the multidisciplinary team.

Signs of Stress

There are often many subtle signs and indicators of stress that are communicated through the body that we may observe in a variety of ways which will have an impact on learning and coping. It may be:

- agitation;
- confusion;
- not wanting to take part, avoiding activities, or following instructions;
- withdrawing from engagement;
- reduced focus and concentration;
- tiredness, even exhaustion, difficulty sleeping;
- frustration which may be displayed as increased or escalating behaviours;
- sadness;
- the complete opposite – loud, boisterous, and very distracting behaviours. Often interrupting, seeking attention, repeatedly asking questions.

There are also likely to be changes in the body. These include physical symptoms, such as:

- increasing heartbeat, perhaps rapid breathing;
- sweating;
- shaking, or trembling a little;
- complexion may become pale if not sweating or they may be clammy;
- feeling dizzy, uptight and tensions throughout the body, even nausea;
- complaints of a tummy ache, body language may change and become hunched or curled;
- sensory experiences and issues may be heightened or may be lessened and lowered.

Emotions may be experienced, such as:

- feeling worried;
- being irritable;
- exhibiting anger;
- being less patient, sometimes feeling sad, being upset or crying.

This may be exhibited through:

- » fidgeting;
- » becoming loud, or, conversely, isolating oneself from others, avoiding different situations, perhaps becoming withdrawn and uninterested;
- » avoiding looking towards the person talking and definitely avoiding any eye contact, which can feel very uncomfortable;
- » self-harm;
- » feeling the need to get out, 'escape', and to run.

Less obvious could be changes to their thoughts, and the information that they are processing. They may find it very difficult to focus or concentrate, have feelings of inner fear and panic, worry about doing something wrong, yet be too scared to ask for help. They may have difficulty retaining information, listening, and following instructions, and this will have an impact on their ability to learn.

For many young people these feelings may be infrequent and short lived but when young people have prolonged anxiety it can influence the process of learning.

As reflexologists, we may not be able to solve the reason for anxiety, but we provide a 'whole' therapy experience that starts with the R E C I P E, complemented by the nurturing touch, which will encourage calmness and relaxation, helping that young person to be present in the moment and feel good within and about themselves.

The Influence of Stress on the Nervous System

It is a scientific fact that the nervous system and the endocrine system (along with many other systems) are influenced by high levels of stress, anxiety, anger, and tension and also that the receptiveness of individuals to learning situations and to some demands placed upon them may be restricted or hindered when such states manifest themselves in the body. In the long term, this will have a significant impact for the balance of the frontal lobe of the brain.

Two of the four distinct parts of the cerebral cortex are the frontal and temporal lobes. These comprise the centre for reasoning, problem solving, focus, processing information from the senses, and the management of emotions. Also important is the limbic system, containing the amygdala, which plays a vital role in controlling various emotional behaviours, such as fear, rage, stress, and anxiety.

A lot of information exists about this area, and about how the structures within play a role in learning and managing emotions. There are many approaches within the world of reflexology and, although his approach differs significantly from my own, I find Hamish Edgar's work very interesting and you may find it worth following up. He is an established reflexology tutor and explains in his book *Limbic Reflexology* (2016) – the approach he founded – that 'the main role of the complex networks of the limbic brain is to continually monitor and respond to both external, and internal environments'. Edgar continues by saying that 'The limbic brain is where much processing takes place and where our responses are largely determined'. This sentence alone should encourage you to consider the importance of the regulatory process in the limbic system and how this may influence a young person's responses and emotional regulation to allow them to manage to receive new information and engage in learning.

There is much support that we can offer through our individual experience and crafted skills of reflexology. But, for me, it is not necessarily just about the techniques that is important, it is also about the framework around our touch time and, very importantly, it is also about the method of delivery that gives the body time to gather the information that we are communicating.

Gathering and Processing Information

Not only do we gather information in different ways, we also gather it at varied rates and speeds, and process and respond at different speeds. When we experience the environment and particular situations, we gather information through our many sensory modalities, to build our unique view of the world around us in different ways.

I am going to mention the term sensory processing disorder (SPD). You may know SPD by the more recent name 'sensory processing difficulties'. The initial name, using the word 'disorder', is used less today in the UK – we tend to use the word 'difficulty' – but it is still used in the USA. It is also used in *The Out-of-Sync Child*, by Carol Stock Kranowitz (2022); I value the information in the book, but this just highlights my previous allusion to the use of names, labels and terms and that what sits comfortably with you might not with someone else.

Sensory processing and information processing difficulties mean that a person may have problems regulating and coping with responses and seek further, or hide from, stimuli. It does not refer to one difficulty but covers a variety that may co-occur.

Kranowitz gives a brief definition of SPD as 'the inability to use information received through the senses in order to function smoothly in daily life'.

It used to be generally thought that there were five senses, but it is now recognised that there are many more. I usually think about these eight, but you might add more:

- » sight (visual);
- » taste (gustatory);
- » touch (somatosensory) – giving touch and being touched;
- » hearing (auditory);
- » smell (olfactory);
- » vestibular (balance)
- » proprioceptive (movement and awareness of where our limbs may be and how our bodies move);
- » interoceptive (how we feel inside, and this may determine how we respond to the information we have gathered).

Once the central nervous system (CNS) gathers information through the senses it then needs to be interpreted and made sense of so that the body can respond. And it's important to know that the senses gather the information differently at different stages of a young person's development.

Once we have started to gather information through all our senses, we rely on how the information is then interpreted, made sense of, and responded to; we all take different times to work with information that we collect and different times to respond – our brains work differently.

Although we are all different, many of the young people with diverse and complex needs experience differences and some difficulties with the way they gather the messages and the time needed to respond to the information. This can be addressed by reflexologists when they take time to consider the delivery of the touch through the FRT method and allow sufficient time for the body to process the information of that touch.

For example, it may be that the person you are supporting has difficulty with auditory processing, which could result in poor perception of speech and sounds. They may have visual processing difficulties, and may need good visual aids to support the information you are sharing, and/or a difficulty with awareness. Diane Hudson sets this out really clearly in her book, *Specific Learning Difficulties* (2015) when she says 'some people are described as having a slow processing speed and so will take longer to absorb information and think about a response, the interpretation of the information takes longer'.

Hudson goes on to say that 'students with slow processing speed will, therefore benefit from having extra time'. For me, this statement is important, for extra time to gather and process all information must include that extra time is given for the body to gather the information from the touch of the reflexologist. This is why the FRT framework asks the reflexologist to consider the method of delivery to reduce the amount of information we provide through our touch.

We know that the information and messages that are gathered by receptors and neurons are transmitted to the brain, which responds by signalling a release of neurotransmitters or chemicals. What is important here is that you are aware of the diverse needs of your young clients who may have difficulties taking in, making sense of, responding to, and even remembering the information you are providing to them, so you need to have a toolkit of strategies and communication methods available.

The delivery of reflexology using the protocol of FRT can support your therapy. It uses increased repetition, reducing change by using a smaller number of techniques so as not to overwhelm the body with information and gives the body time to gather the information with the intent to calm, relax, and rebalance, subduing or quietening the release of cortisol, which helps to support the balance of the frontal lobe.

'Happy' Chemicals

There are many 'happy' chemicals that positive touch encourages the body to release. These, of course, all play a vital role as they work in harmony, and I know if I briefly mention dopamine, serotonin, endorphins, and oxytocin, you will all probably begin to think about how they act to support a positive mood when they are released, but it is the release of oxytocin that I am going to focus upon.

Stress, anxiety, and worries trigger the hormone cortisol. When the amygdala detects a threat and processes fear, it sends signals to other areas in the brain which can cause the release of cortisol from the adrenals.

Cortisol is just one hormone that is involved in the fight, flight, or freeze response. It is, of course, a necessary hormone but, if it is released at high and long-term levels, it can be damaging, as long-term chronic levels have been shown to actively corrode learning connections within the brain. If we extrapolate from this that elevated levels through ongoing high levels of anxiety will impair learning, schools should be thinking about how to set up a learning environment that will be less stressful and look at support through therapeutic interventions to help young people manage better during the school day. This links to the comment noted by Beardon earlier in this chapter.

Barbara and Kevin Kunz in their book, *Reflexology for Children* (1996) interestingly state that 'using reflexology techniques to provide relaxation helps the body break up particular patterns of stress. The stress thus does not accumulate to cause wear and tear on the body'. Here, it is the word 'accumulation' that is important.

Oxytocin is a naturally occurring neurochemical (sometimes called a neuropeptide or a neurotransmitter, produced in the hypothalamus, deep in the mid-brain) that acts like a hormone in our bodies, meaning it crosses the blood–brain barrier and circulates in the bloodstream as well as in the brain, to regulate the arousal level of our nervous system. Oxytocin is released through touch, warmth, and affectionate connection.

Any warm, loving, touch can release oxytocin – hugs, snuggles, holding hands, massage, and body work. Neuroscience has confirmed that because of how our brains process information, even thinking about someone who loves us or someone we deeply care for is enough to activate the release of oxytocin in the brain.

It is suggested that augmenting the release of oxytocin can help the body and mind to calm and it is very interesting that Professor Kerstin Uvnas-Moberg, in *The Oxytocin Factor* (2003), suggests that since oxytocin reduces stress, increasing its release within the body can improve opportunities for learning.

So, if your young clients are enjoying the whole therapy session and there is an increase in the release of oxytocin and an increase in the feel-good factor, ask yourself at the end of the therapy session, are they leaving the therapy room in a better frame of mind than when they arrived? Are they returning to the classroom better able to take part in activities and also allow learning to take place? Remember, this is about the efficacy of your therapy session during the school day.

Studies and Research

There are very few studies available to validate the benefits of reflexology for young people with additional, complex, and diverse needs, particularly the benefits to offering this therapeutic intervention on the timetable during the school day. We are beginning to collect information from FRT reflexologists and senior management within the schools where it is part of the timetable, but there is a wealth of information about the benefits of massage.

My book would not be complete without sharing the work of Tiffany Field (Director of the Touch Research Institutes, University of Miami School of Medicine and Nova South-eastern University, USA) and her amazing book *Touch Therapy* (Field, 2000). I draw your attention particularly to a chapter on enhancing attentiveness with a study supporting young people with attention deficit hyperactivity disorder (ADHD) and autism. (I will just add that I really dislike the use of the word 'disorder' and the times are changing.)

Field states:

> Attention deficits like Autism and Attention Deficit Disorder in some children are very disruptive of classroom behaviour and learning. Very little is known about the aetiology of these disorders, but some behavioural management and some arousal-reducing therapies like massage seem to have positive effects.
>
> Although most study samples seem to have been quite small in number the touch activities have been regular and consistent. They have shown that the touch therapy alleviated anxiety and decreased cortisol levels and depression in child psychiatric patients (Field et al., 2000).

Field went on to state that vagal activity increased during touch therapy and, since that study, vagal activity has been associated with increased attention span (Porges, 1991). Touch therapy may reduce the off-task behaviour noted in autistic children.

One study of 22 preschool children (12 boys) with autism investigated the effects of touch therapy on three problems commonly associated with autism: inattentiveness (off-task behaviour), touch aversion, and withdrawal. The results opened much discussion that both groups within the study improved on some behaviours, but that there was increased attentiveness noted during classroom observations, not something we can go into discussion with here, but very interesting patterns of change following touch therapies.

I also refer to a book titled *Clinical Reflexology: A Guide for Health Professionals*, edited by Peter Mackereth and Denise Tiran (2002), for a chapter by Evelyn Gale ('Advocating the use of reflexology for people with a learning disability') who, at the time, was a lecturer in nursing at Keele University. The focus of her PhD was an investigation into the use of touch by nurses and its effects on people with a learning disability, advocating the use of reflexology.

Gale's points are very valuable. I think her work, suggestions, and early guidelines raised a lot of awareness and have given inspiration, encouragement, and confidence to many reflexologists, myself included. It is interesting that she concludes that 'reflexology is increasingly and enthusiastically being introduced to the care of people with learning disabilities and provides a valuable therapeutic tool', but she recognises that although feedback and studies show many positives, more contemporary and related investigations are needed. This is an area that to this day still requires more investigation, and one, I think you will agree, that is very difficult to establish within this field.

I was delighted when I recently came across a study titled 'Research of Hand Reflexology Stimulation in Children with ADHD' that was presented to the Annual International Conference on Cognitive-Social and Behavioural Sciences (2020). Researchers Lavrinĉík and Tománková from the Czech Republic undertook experimental research with children aged 6–9, diagnosed with ADHD, noting that motoric disorders frequently co-occurred with this condition. They were looking at the difficulties the children so affected might experience in trying to perform common practical tasks associated with the learning process (e.g., drawing, IT, etc.).

The aim of the study was to investigate whether improvement of fine and gross motor skills could be improved through the application of hand reflexology therapy. It concluded that there was a significant improvement and that further research should be conducted to see if the methodology employed with this group could be beneficial to other disadvantageous conditions, such as cerebral palsy.

It is perhaps important to consider that the improvement in motor skills through reflexology stimulation and the realisation this gave to each of those young people as to their potential would increase the release of oxytocin, the feel-good factor, and support their emotional well-being. An improvement in control of motor coordination and awareness of their personal ability will indeed raise self-esteem.

For me, it is reassuring that research is looking at using the skilful delivery of reflexology as an approach that adds valuable support.

Chapter 6: Emotional Well-being, Consent, and Connection

I am sure you will agree with me that securing consent from each young person that you invite for reflexology is vital. No matter how enthusiastic parents and carers may be, or how keen teachers are for the young person in their class to receive your touch, or how enthusiastic you are as the reflexologist knowing its many benefits, this is not sufficient on its own.

Never Assume

Everyone needs to be given a voice to consent. But what exactly does it mean and how do you ascertain consent when supporting young people with learning difficulties, with communication difficulties, with profound and multiple learning difficulties, with very few or no words?

Being in control is a significant part of our well-being and our right. First, be clear about what consent means straight from a dictionary: 'Permission for something to happen or agreement to do something'.

The Process

From a practical point of view, in schools where reflexology supported by the FRT Framework is used, a referral form is usually available in the staff room, on the server, or direct from the reflexologist. This means that teachers can consider the potential of the therapy session and how it may support their learners. Along with tick boxes there is also space for staff to add any other comments and/or questions. Together we discuss how the session may offer the best support and if the young person being referred will benefit from:

- » relaxation and a sense of calm 'in the moment';
- » the easing of discomfort and tension;
- » having anxious or low feelings alleviated;
- » an opportunity to share feelings, meaningful communication time;

- » building a new 1:1 relationship through positive touch activities;
- » being in control and raising awareness of consent, giving permission for positive touch on feet and/or hands, building confidence;
- » support for some individual learning targets;
- » improvement to their general well-being and, if relevant, having some health issues highlighted by parents addressed.

Then the reflexologist provides:

- » a consent form for parents/carers to complete (although consent is ongoing and independently given by the young person coming along for the session even when consent is given by the parent/carer);
- » a short questionnaire for home;
- » a short questionnaire for classroom teacher and support staff.

In 2022 a reflexologist using the FRT framework was welcomed into a school to support young people with the therapy session on their timetable. I was delighted to hear her feedback that the one thing that really impressed the school was the fact that professional documentation and expectations were in place. She could provide the school with guidelines for reflexology which could be developed and edited to meet that school's needs and expectations. *This documentation, as previously noted in Chapter 4, is available to all reflexologists who attend the FRT training course.*

The reflexologist will receive the consent form from the parents/carers keen for their child to be offered the opportunity to receive reflexology. Consent is ongoing and it can be retracted at any point by parents, but, most importantly, it is led and can be retracted by the young person themselves.

I cannot state this often enough, and as you will notice I do repeat it, the ongoing process is very much a pupil-led activity. It is they who are in control, and they have the option to receive or not to receive. It is up to the reflexologist to involve the young person as much as possible as they work together to make sure the young person understands what is being offered and shows and gives their approval.

You will see in the stories later that consent is requested in a variety of ways with different methods of communication. Ido Kedar refers to the absolute importance of having a voice in whatever medium and with whatever support is appropriate when he writes in his book, *Ido in Autismland* 'Language is our pathway to connecting deeply with others. To be denied communication is to limit one to a life of frustration, loneliness and being misunderstood'.

Much more recently, as I was bringing this information together, a series titled *Inside Our Autistic Minds* was aired on BBC2, presented by Chris Packham, who is is autistic, a naturalist, presenter, and author. In the series, he helps autistic people illustrate how their minds work, giving them a voice through a variety of methods of meaningful communication, helping them to connect with their family and friends and bringing such valuable information to the public.

As I explored in the previous chapter, the body and mind use up a lot of energy through worry and fear of uncertain situations. When our emotional balance is unstable in the long term, the sympathetic nervous system is working in overdrive, and it can become easily overwhelmed and exhausted through trying to communicate. It is necessary to be aware of what could happen if a person is not listened to or understood, and we just assume we know best.

Martin Pistorius, the author of *Ghost Boy* (2011), shares his experience about the horror and then the disappointment he felt when he realised he would spend the rest of his life as powerlessly as he lived each of his days and eventually he says, 'I didn't try to respond or react but stared at the world with blank expression'.

With regard to consent, we can accept 'implied consent', which is when the behaviour, signals, sounds, movements, or stillness of the person we are working with is interpreted to help with the decision making.

You will read about the stillness and quietness having a meaning in Fred's story. As much as I would love all my young people to attend for reflexology, if they don't perhaps they are having a difficult day, maybe they are just not in the mood, maybe it is something else, but they just do not want to come along! As practitioners, we must try our best to interpret their communication to ensure that we meet their wishes, and never to assume or presume you know what is right or what they want.

The Mental Capacity Act 2005 provides a statutory framework for people who lack the capacity to make decisions for themselves and does support the term 'implied consent'.

Think about the FRT RECIPE and how you can create an environment to provide the opportunity for consent to be given or not given and the decision respected.

How Do the Sessions Run?

Not only is it essential and respectful to ask for consent, but we can only do this if sufficient information, using appropriate and meaningful methods of communication, and sufficient time for response are in place. I wonder how often you might just assume that it's okay and off you go. The FRT framework and RECIPE asks you to consider, think, and act on what you need to have in place to alleviate anxiety a little and begin to support emotional well-being, self-esteem, and respect before your touch. Hirstwood and Gray (1995), in their book *A Practical Guide to the Use of Multi-sensory Rooms*, write, 'all too often people are taken to places and activities without knowing where they are going, who is taking them and what the activity is'.

There are numerous methods and approaches that are available to help to make your communication more appropriate and meaningful. Think about the RECIPE, be respectful, be empathetic, learn about effective communication methods, prepare yourself and the person you are supporting and allow sufficient time, then evaluate and reflect on how effective you have been and how you can work together to make it better and possibly easier.

Meaningful Communication

Imagine how you might feel if you were in a wheelchair, and someone began pushing it without acknowledging you or letting you know what they were going to do or even that they were there, as noted earlier in this chapter by Hirstwood and Gray. Imagine being focused and taking part in something and suddenly being led/redirected and not knowing what was going to be happening. Wouldn't you need time to prepare yourself?

As you will see in the stories from the therapy, there are many different approaches to support, and it is important to find the right support to make the connection meaningful. This can include social stories, objects of reference, eye gaze, use of tablets such as iPad, signs, symbols, visual timetables, photographs, and, most important of all, allowing sufficient time to help the young person to understand what is going to be happening and help them to prepare for the activity. This helps to alleviate some anxiety before the touch of reflexology but remember that communication doesn't stop at the therapy door.

Carol Gray initiated and developed the use of social stories in the early 1990s. Social stories can be used (although may not be right for everyone) to help provide meaningful information and provide an understanding of an event or an action, giving a short description of a particular situation, which helps a person to understand what to expect and, thereby, reduce anxiousness/anxiety a little. A social story can also be used to acknowledge achievements, so, for reflexology, it could show all the things and activities that they have enjoyed and the routine of the whole session at the end.

A social story is not complicated, it needs to be short and clear to help to provide some information that is meaningful, as I did for George.

I created four stories, each one of which could be used at different times of the session, and they have a different amount of information written in clear short sentences. They may have just photos, just text, hand drawn pictures, or both text and illustrative material. My four stories are used to explain the following.

1. What is foot reflexology?
2. Why do I have reflexology?
3. Going for reflexology.
4. What happens in the reflexology therapy room?

The stories are printed in A4 size and are used for as many sessions as necessary. The story below was used for the first four sessions to help George to become comfortable with the routine of going to the therapy room and to know he had a choice as to whether or not to accept the invitation.

Here is an example of story number 3, 'Going for reflexology'.

Lorraine is the name of the reflexologist.

Lorraine wears a purple polo shirt.

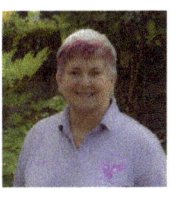

Lorraine will come to the classroom to meet George when it is time to go for reflexology.

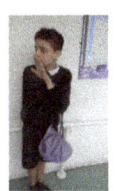

George can choose to carry the reflexology bag. The bag has a picture of a hand and foot on it.

George and Lorraine will walk together to the reflexology room.

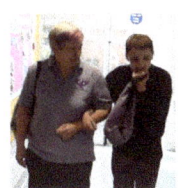

There is a photograph of Lorraine on the door of the reflexology room.

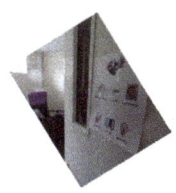

George, do you want to go for reflexology?

George really took to using the FRT toolkit. It was a valuable object of reference. He would usually carry it over one arm or hold it and swing it along as we walked to the therapy room.

Supporting with cues such as social stories, prompts, photos, and symbols, as I mentioned previously, may be important and we may use a visual timetable or a communication strip. You will see these used in the storyboard and in Harry's story.

Naoki Higashida, in his book *The Reason I Jump: One Boy's Voice from the Silence of Autism*, tries to work out for himself why they are needed. (The book is formatted as questions that Naoki asks of himself and his answers.) Naoki says,

> I don't really know why people with autism need cues, but I know that I'm one of them. Since we already know what we'll be doing next, surely we should just be able to get on with it, unprompted, right? Yes I think so too! But the fact is, doing the action without the cue can be really, really tough.

It is interesting that he also suggests in his book that we should support cues and visuals to 'talk through the day's plan'. I have created a visual board which is available for prompts and cues in my therapy room, with which I always also use verbal support and often gesture and pointing.

It may be different in each school, but in my school each session comprises more than just the touch of reflexology. I pencil in 30 minutes or, for some sessions, 40 minutes on the timetable. This allows for:

- » collection from the classroom;
- » travel to the therapy room;
- » arrival and preparation;
- » up to 20 minutes of touch time (20 minutes is the maximum);
- » preparation to finish, which must not be underestimated;
- » travel back to class or to the next activity.

Then a few minutes is needed to check that the room is ready for the next young person. Perhaps something needs to be moved, or some symbols should be removed from the wall to make it meaningful for the next client, or music should be put on or turned off, depending on whether or not it helps them to recognise the session. I quickly check my notes from the previous session to see whether there is anything I need to consider and then go along to the next young person.

What happens if the young person does not want to stay for 20 minutes? I may try to encourage them to stay a little longer, depending on what is going on, but ultimately it is their decision. I might say that the teacher may be disappointed that we are returning earlier than he/she may have anticipated! I say this only because I have been there and done that with my teacher's hat on, and if you have the opportunity for one pupil in your class to be off enjoying another activity it allows you more time with others. But it doesn't always work that way.

That's why, when you are welcomed into a school, it's worth being clear about your plans and expectations for the sessions and what might happen if you do return after only a few minutes.

I recall one young lady whom I had been working with for ten sessions who, one day, decided that she didn't want to go into the therapy room any more. She enjoyed the walk from the classroom and she seemed to enjoy the interaction along the way; she had very few words and used some symbols for communication. But when she stood still at the door and didn't move forwards, that told me that, for whatever reason, she was choosing to end her sessions.

My records do highlight that, as we only had three weeks until the end of the term, I did try for those weeks, but it became a walk, a stop, and then a walk back and I never was able to ascribe any meaning to her decision. She didn't seem unhappy, and she seemed to enjoy the sessions for the first ten weeks. Could she have been masking a feeling that it was expected that she took part?

Let's talk about masking, or camouflaging. These are terms used to describe a practice that many young people who are autistic may use, perhaps feeling that something is expected of them even though they may not like it or might feel uncomfortable. If, indeed, the young person mentioned above was making herself go into the session and tolerate the touch, this could increase anxiety and have the opposite effect to that which was intended.

Maybe, after the first ten sessions, she felt comfortable enough to say 'I don't like it' or' I don't want it any more' through her actions. Being respectful of choice is paramount, as is understanding and using alternative methods of communication to meet an individual's needs. This little sentence popped out for me in Martin Pistorious's *Ghost Boy*: 'What is the point in learning to communicate if no one will listen'.

I have some smiley photos and video clips of the young lady in the therapy room. Her parents felt that it was a happy smile, so we are not sure why it changed. I will never know what the issue was, but the important thing to highlight here is having the consent of the person receiving the therapy and their right to say no thank you and be listened to respectfully.

How can you learn about masking? Possibly through educational acceptance that it exists, experience, and being open to neurodiversity and discussion, where possible, about how people are feeling and how they feel they 'have to behave' and why.

How Many Sessions?

Through discussion with the headteacher in your school you will decide how many sessions you feel would be good to pencil in. Consider that it may take time:

- » to visit a new part of the school;
- » for a client to feel comfortable with a new person in their life;
- » for them to accept the touch;
- » to allow themselves to relax;
- » to increase the length of the sessions (you will notice in one of the case studies the increase of touch time from 2 minutes to 14 minutes over a 20-week period).

Through discussions with my school, we decided on the round figure of 20 weeks, to allow time for all of the above.

Feedback

Just like the repetition of your touch, the sessions and the structure become familiar and you can hope that 20 weeks allows enough time to see changes and responses. You will get comments and feedback from staff and parents as they begin to recognise and observe responses.

As the end of the 20 sessions nears, I begin to complete my report and discuss with the class teacher and the headteacher if the sessions should come to an end or continue. You will see in George's story that the weekly session became part of his timetable for seven years!

I do get asked how much feedback may be useful. Typically, I will provide updates to staff half-termly (that's every six to seven weeks), and similarly to parents, but only if there is something significant I feel I need to share. Feedback may be in the form of a short written summary, and photos are always well received, as are brief video clips. It's great to be able to show and share what happens in the therapy room. Occasionally, a feedback phone call to parents, though I don't do this very often. It's worth mentioning here that I think it is important to maintain regular follow-ups with staff, and for them to know they can approach me with queries and comments at any time.

I will take the opportunity to mention photos and videos for reasons of safety, well-being, and accountability. My initial consent form asks for permission for these to be taken in the therapy room, particularly as we work with most of our young people on a 1:1 basis.

Video recording is very useful and can prove valuable if something unusual occurs or if a situation changes very quickly; sometimes unexpected situations can take us by surprise. It can offer me the chance to follow up and reflect on my actions, even listening to the wording I might have used – a very good learning and supportive tool for both myself and the young person. I do not have time to watch all the videos but, if necessary, I can take a look and pop a note on to the record sheet. But usually, it suffices to share the work in the therapy room.

I recall one such occasion where the video was very helpful. It was a session in 2012, which I thought was going well. The young person was calm, he had made the decision that day to have the green blanket and chose to have the music on. All was delightful until, 12 minutes in, just as if a switch had been flipped, he became very unsettled, sat upright, and became very anxious. I tried to calm him by speaking with a soft, soothing voice, to no avail.

Of course, my initial thought was 'what have I done wrong!' I became slightly anxious in those few seconds while trying to work out the best way to help, during which he became quite distressed and started to knock over whatever he could to get out of the way, including me. He needed to get out of the room quickly, so I picked up his socks and shoes. This was not a time for asking questions. He walked, I followed. Fortunately, we went in the direction of his classroom. It is not advisable to walk barefoot through the corridors and not something that is usually allowed, but if you are someone reading this who is supporting young people who may have a meltdown episode, the best thing to do is to support from a safe distance and give them space. By the time we were nearer to the classroom he seemed a little calmer, but still unsettled. He took time in his space and then allowed a member of staff to help him with his shoes; he seemed quite tired.

When I felt brave enough to share the video the next day with the member of staff, 12 minutes in she said, 'Hear the lawn mower being turned on?' Yes, there was grass cutting happening just outside the therapy room! With hypersensitive hearing and a real dislike of that sound, this was indeed the switch that caused him to become so distressed.

That was a learning curve in more ways than one. First, I felt relieved that it wasn't something I could have avoided! However, I felt sad that it was an action that caused such immediate distress. Second, I felt reassured that I had coped in an appropriate way, although I used too much language and asked too many questions in the first few seconds of his actions. The conversation with staff really helped me should a similar experience occur in the future.

This gives me the opportunity to bring to your attention the term 'autistic meltdown'. I understand it as a term for an expression of immense distress, as in the case of the young man above. He was communicating to me the need to get away from the challenging situation, which I did not recognise.

A 'meltdown' is very different to getting annoyed, having a tantrum, or a strop; it is being completely overwhelmed by the situation. If you are a reflexologist looking to support young people that are autistic, it is advisable to learn as much as possible, to observe in class, and discuss with staff what strategies they would advise to best manage meltdowns to help ensure safety for you and the person you are supporting. The best thing is for these stressful situations not to occur at all, but they do, and may be, as in the example above, completely out of our control, so please take advice from staff and don't be afraid to ask questions.

Prompts, photos, and symbols, such as I mentioned earlier, *will not* be helpful during a meltdown. There are many other ways you can offer support, from staying back, allowing space and being quiet to giving a hug and verbal reassurance, but you will need to know this is different for each person.

Bringing together much of the information shared so far in this book, now join me as I invite you to the therapy room.

Chapter 7: An Invitation to the Therapy Room

I FEEL I have already talked a lot about the success and many benefits of integrating reflexology, supported by the FRT framework, into the school day, and I have already emphasised a few times about the importance that getting to know a young person carries. The RECIPE highlights how it is not just about working with the clients, but about building meaningful connections beyond the touch, and every element of the session needs to be considered to achieve success.

I draw inspiration from something said by Brene Brown, an American professor and author, in her book, *Atlas of the Heart* (2021), that is important whether you are a reflexologist, teacher, or parent or carer reading this: 'Connection is the energy that exists between people when they feel seen, heard, and valued. … And when they derive sustenance and strength from the relationship'.

There is some lovely text from Mary Atkinson, an award-winning complementary therapist, in her book, *Healing Touch for Children*, which really resonates with my work. In this book, she looks at the many benefits of touch and I really like how she uses the term 'respectful touch', which, she points out, 'can help induce a calm atmosphere and attentive learning'.

Presenting a Case Study

A case study is usually written to provide the reader with clear, structured data about a particular process where the person/people taking part are anonymous.

I deliberated for many months about sharing our work together and how best to do this. I questioned using photos and names – was I exploiting the confidentiality of the therapy room? And, in sharing such information far and wide, would this open an opportunity for negative comments? What did I feel I would gain by using photos and the real names of real people?

I refer to a recent article in the PMLD Link (Profound and Multiple Learning Difficulties) magazine by Joanna Grace. Jo is a doctoral researcher, sensory engagement and inclusion specialist, and founder of The Sensory Projects. The article was published as I was completing the first draft of my book which raised this very point; it resonated with the thought process I had been going through and she was able to put it much more eloquently than I, but it was all about my worries. The title of the article is 'Share their picture, say their name. Is it safe to share photos of people with profound intellectual and multiple disabilities online? The ethics of being presented to the online world' (Grace, 2022). And although she is talking about the online world, I know this book will go out in print as well as on social media platforms.

I asked similar questions of myself and the wonderful young people who feature in the book. The response I received was so reassuring. Parents began to thank me for the opportunity for this to be a platform for their children to celebrate themselves and to share information about how they cope with and manage some of their difficulties. Joanna Grace suggests that visibility matters and that, by showing and sharing, the public can become more aware, prejudice may be slowly dissolved, and we can challenge, if necessary, any responses.

For the purposes of this book, the reflexology FRT framework report and data collection serve as a platform to share stories from the therapy room and share information that you may find interesting for further research.

Much of my evidence relies on observation, particularly capturing facial expressions and some gestures for those who are not able verbalise their feelings and responses. I'm so proud that using photos offers an opportunity to the young people to show and share their joy in their own way.

Each story will be presented in a similar way, albeit with some variations. Some will include more details, while others will have fewer and occasionally there will be additional significant information. But, despite the differences, the overall framework used is consistent and the main purpose and intention of each session remains the same. I will:

- » Introduce the participant.
- » Detail the teacher and staff referral.
- » Encourage you to consciously consider the FRT R E C I P E.
- » Detail the classroom observation: what I noticed and advice I was given.
- » Provide my Reflexology Reflection with insights from my records.
- » Explore some general information.
- » Consider Efficacy and Effectiveness: What worked and what didn't.
- » Share feedback from the teachers, parents/carers and/or participants.
- » Share tips for reflexologists with key considerations.
- » Include links and articles for further reading.
- » Offer my closing thoughts of gratitude and learning.

I am immensely proud to share these very personal stories to highlight the value that the therapeutic intervention of reflexology, supported by the FRT framework, brings during the school day. So, it is only right that we extend an invitation to you to join us in the therapy room, where we can share our experiences and you can feel the effectiveness of our connection and the value it brings.

Chapter 8: Meet George

'I like both feet worked at the same time, I tell Lorraine with a gentle kick.'

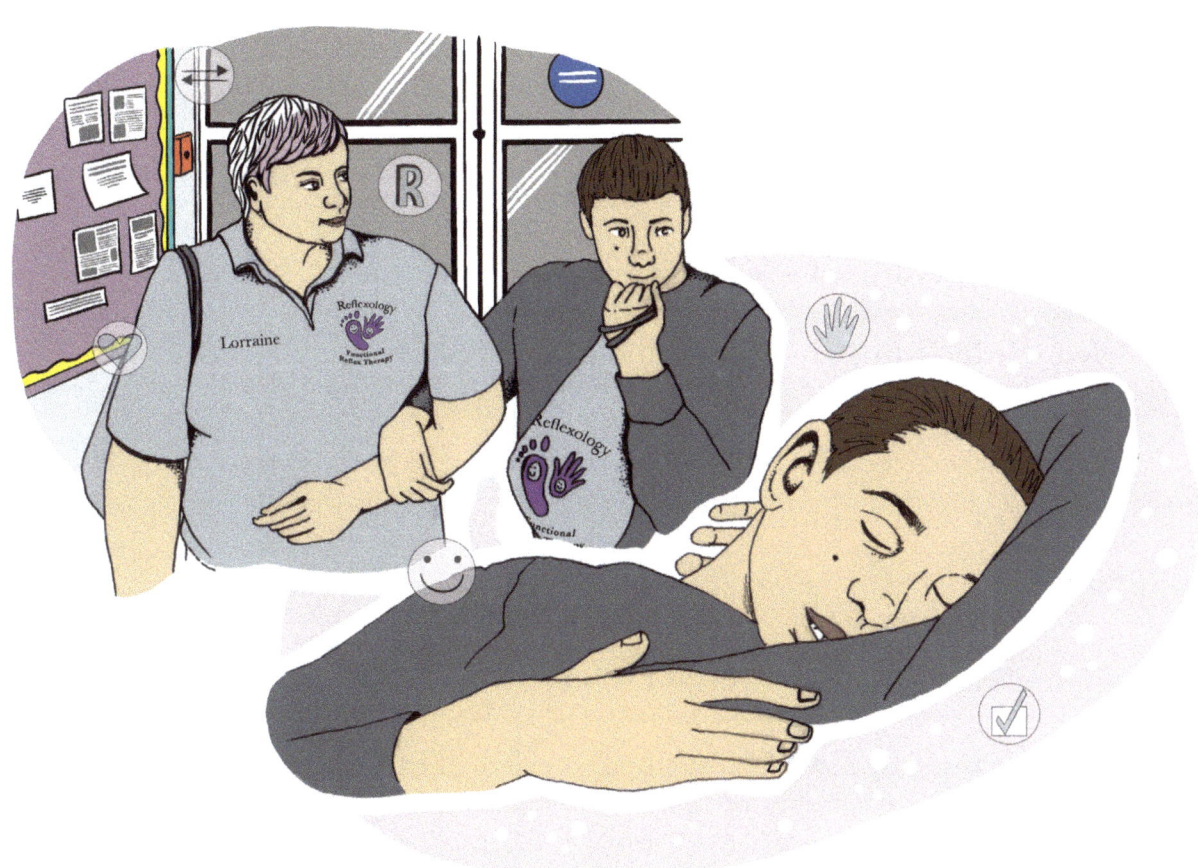

OUR WORK TOGETHER began in September 2012 when George was 11 years of age, and subsequently I had the privilege to invite George for reflexology for seven years as a weekly therapy session on his timetable.

George has a great smile, lots of energy and is usually very active, loving the movement and rhythm that sitting on the large therapy ball can provide. He is autistic, with intellectual and communication difficulties, and a condition named Schwachman-Diamond syndrome that affects many parts of the body, particularly the bone marrow, pancreas, and skeletal system.

The Process

Teacher referral

At the time of the referral, George was having quite a few days away from school as he was prone to challenges with his health. The teacher wondered if this may have added to his anxiousness and contribute to his unsettledness. She said, 'George would often fret and could be agitated. He regularly seemed very uptight and tense, needing time to regulate to gather and process information.'

And she noted that George would often find the noise around him unsettling, which could make it difficult for him to cope and focus on tasks. The team around George was already offering him time out and regular breaks but noted he was often frustrated, and this showed itself with him getting quite distressed. Sometimes he had flare-ups with a skin condition, which also caused discomfort and irritation, reducing his ability to focus and join in with activities.

The teacher wanted him to:

- experience time away from the busyness of the classroom;
- begin to feel more comfortable moving around the school and into new areas, as he could be very anxious when visiting somewhere unfamiliar;
- develop a new relationship and become familiar and comfortable with, and trusting of, a new member of staff;
- receive the positive touch therapy, accept the touch, and show calmness and relaxation from receiving it;
- indicate enjoyment of the session when returning to the classroom.

Classroom observation

Observing George gave me the opportunity to watch and listen to the clear, concise, meaningful communication and interaction between the staff and George, which was very helpful.

He used very few words, and there were a variety of methods of communication available for use within the classroom, but he found it difficult to express his thoughts and feelings other than through behaviour that, at times, could be challenging for him and for those around him.

I listened to the vocabulary and how the staff addressed George, so I could be consistent. I came away feeling I needed to develop clear information to help George to know what was going to happen, which might alleviate some of his anxiety before my touch of reflexology. This would allow the session to run more smoothly and be more meaningful.

After taking the opportunity to chat with the speech and language therapist (SLT), I decided to put together a social story and she reassured me that it would be useful to him.

Before the touch

I provided a photograph of myself and the FRT toolkit that could be added to his visual timetable. (More information about a visual timetable can be found in Cedric's story.)

I also designed a social story. An example is shown in Chapter 6.

During the touch

I noted George's sensitivity to noise, so I had to think about how I would set up and create the right space for him.

I reduced arousal levels in the therapy room, ensured it was a quiet environment, ascertaining his consent for music or no music, his preferred choice for type of music, and allowed sufficient time for transition and to gather and respond to instruction. This information helped with the success of the session.

Visual cues using photographs and symbols, objects of reference from the FRT toolkit, helped him to recognise the structure for the session, and again the designated space that had been created allowed him time to respond.

It was very important for me to bear in mind the importance of communication: the gestures, the tone of my voice, so that, even if George was not listening to a specific verbal instruction, he would be aware of my tone, my body posture and positioning. It was important to consider approaching him from the side or crouching down rather than looking down from an overpowering position.

It was essential to provide a comfortable space and an enjoyable sensory experience, increasing the release of oxytocin, thus helping to subdue cortisol levels, offering the opportunity and time to calm tension within his mind and body.

George seemed to enjoy all the movements; at no point did he ever remove his feet but when I worked on just one foot at a time, he cheekily used to give me a little kick with the other foot as if to say 'I like both feet worked at the same time.' Although I never presumed that was the case and tested it briefly in many sessions, when I adapted my techniques to work both feet at the same time throughout the session, he seemed calm, usually made happy sounds and giggles, and stopped kicking my hands.

Being an active listener and knowing behaviour is a form of communication, I needed to interpret the kick! When I started bringing my work together, I was not aware of this book, but I recently read Tony Osgood's *Supporting Positive Behaviour in Intellectual Disabilities and Autism: Practical Strategies for Addressing Challenging Behaviour* (2020), in which he refers to being an active listener. This is a term that I have been using for many years and he describes it as: 'Active listening means taking not only what is said at face value – a literal interpretation – but also what is meant. To listen actively we decode words or behaviour into meaning'.

Reflexology and reflection insights from my records

When applying reflexology techniques along the spine reflex, I noted tension in his ankles noticeably decreased. This allowed his feet to naturally turn outwards. Recognising this as one of the movements he most preferred and being able to work on both feet simultaneously (which he loved) it was delivered with much repetition within every session.

23rd January, 2013 – *total touch time 12 minutes*: this was two minutes longer than the previous week's touch time, removed feet, sat up quickly, pinched my arm, wanted to put his socks and shoes on.

You may question whether that pinch was acceptable. In the moment, it was George's way of communicating to me. If I could have chosen a better way for him and for me, I would have preferred that and I am sure he would have, too. Causing discomfort to others is not what he wants to be doing, he just needed to communicate.

In the therapy room at this point I placed a board next to George's chair with a laminated symbol which said 'stop'. Over the next few weeks I showed him how he had control to stop the session with this when he was ready, but it didn't really prove successful. My notes referred to me questioning myself – *Did I continue too long? What did I do differently?* I stayed positive and helped him to finish the session as calmly as possible. I counted down without any touch, preparing him as clearly as possible for the end of the session. I had no idea what he might be thinking about! Possibly nothing to do with me or the session at that moment, as it didn't happen too often.

17th May, 2017 – *total touch time 30 minutes.* He was getting over a very heavy cold, and I had a note from home – *very little sleep this week and congested, quite unsettled.*

When I collected George from class, he was very rushed. I was led quickly (well, more like pulled) by George to get out and to the therapy room. Five minutes in the chair and he was asleep. I had a little extra time available so in the therapy room worked particularly around reflex support: head, ear and chest. He was a little grumpy at being woken up but was a lot calmer and took time to replace his socks. No usual smiles but generally 'happy'. Our walk back to class was less rushed and he chose to sit and rock on the bouncy ball near his desk. The intention? To be in a better frame of mind at the end of the session to help him to manage activities back in the classroom.

24th April, 2019 – *total touch time 20 minutes and 5 minutes self-care support.* He was very comfortable with me, would laugh and enjoy a little banter. Smiles and taking time at the end of the session and at this point beginning to tolerate and take time with the introduction of some self-care techniques to encourage taking time with a squeezing movement and a big breath.

After the touch

Bringing the touch and the therapy session to a close, the routine was always finished with a very specific technique and a clear countdown to communicate the end of our work together. Countdowns are often used within school and signal coming to the end of an activity and a time for change.

George liked to count down with me, although his numbers often got quite quick and I would encourage him to slow down. When he got to know me very well it used to be a bit of fun at the end of the session when I could say, '5 wait, wait, wait, 4 wait, wait, wait, 3 wait, wait, wait ...' – well, I think you get the idea. We used to laugh our way through that.

For George, returning the towel to his toolkit and carrying it back to the classroom helped him finish and transition.

Interestingly, every time we returned to the classroom, although he had enjoyed the session and he returned calmly, he was always quick to signal his finish with me, sometimes with a little gentle push and a gesture towards the door!

Efficacy and effectiveness

I worked with George for over 150 sessions of reflexology. When he first started, he was so anxious he would be in the chair for three or four minutes. Long before we finished working together, he was thoroughly enjoying 20 minutes and was calm enough to sit and replace his socks and shoes, smile and engage with laughter and some great sounds.

When I first worked with him, as noted by the teacher in her referral, he was often away from school with challenges to his health. However, his medication changed, he grew and made progress in many ways in class. He was present much more than absent and, working alongside many other things, I would like to think that the weekly timetabled sessions may have contributed a supportive role in his well-being and wellness.

I introduced the calming solar plexus squeeze that he could administer himself, encouraging him to count up and breathe and count down and breathe, just to slow himself down. In hindsight, I think I should have introduced this at least a year earlier as I feel it might have become something he would have got into the habit of delivering with his own hands.

Feedback

When I look back at my early records, I recall that George attended the first six sessions supported by a member of staff who helped him to settle and allowed him time to become a little used to me as a new person in his life and begin to connect as he became a little more familiar with the structure of the session. He was extremely anxious and insisted that the member staff who came with him sat next to him.

If you are offered a member of staff to support you, they are not there to judge you! You are working as part of a team, so it can be a positive, helpful start. However, it is something that you need to gradually reduce; you want to be in control of that session and, in George's case, one of the targets of the referral was for him to be comfortable with a new member of staff.

Changing the dynamics

Having another person in the therapy room changes the dynamics immensely even if they are not speaking to you. However, you may also get support staff that find it very difficult not to talk and not to make comments, so you need to have clear supportive guidelines for staff, too.

Fortunately for our sessions, the member of staff began to reduce their input, moving away to the other side of the therapy room, then sitting around the corner, then walking with us to the therapy room but not coming in. I also have to say that the first time this happened George was so relaxed that he drifted off to sleep. Can you guess who I told first? We both got very emotional.

The class teacher said, 'Even if George is having an unsettled time during the school day, when you walk into the classroom Lorraine, he always seems pleased to take the toolkit and go to the therapy room.'

Consistency

Consistency for many of our young people is important. Even if it had not been me offering these sessions, the structure and framework would offer that consistency. (See the consistent use of the framework by Amanda and Seema in Chapter 3.)

Throughout the years that I supported George, many of his teaching staff and support staff changed. I felt privileged to be a constant part of his timetable. When I look back at the photos and videos, I see real progress as a meaningful connection developed.

My records show much improvement in his attendance; I wonder how much the regular reflexology sessions contributed, working alongside general medication and his natural growth and development. Who can say? It certainly became a valuable part of his weekly timetable in so many ways and, according to his parents, also a valuable part of family life.

Parent feedback

Always supportive of the sessions, George's mum took the opportunity to come along to the FRT Rainbow Relaxation Workshop for the family.

I'm going to finish George's story with a beautiful letter. I refer to it during my training sessions for reflexologists and it still brings a little tear to my eye. *Something like this would be great for any reflexologist delivering reflexology with the FRT framework and great for any school!*

19.06.2017

Dear Lorraine,

Thank you for George's reflexology report, we were delighted to read about and see the photographs of his therapy sessions. He looks very relaxed and happy, and we certainly know the benefits which these sessions have for him.

We continue to deliver reflexology on George every night as part of his bedtime routine. We always carry this out on his feet as he much prefers this to his hands. George will get his reflexology bag out, and we follow the routine that you kindly showed Tahira when she completed a workshop with you at school. George prompts us to use the count in and countdown to finish. Depending on how tired George is we tailor the time of the session to suit, George sometimes falls asleep during the session but if he is still awake will put his reflexology bag away before settling down for the night. We have seen a significant improvement with how quickly George now goes off to sleep. He also takes a melatonin tablet one hour before bed, but we have found that he needs the combination of this and the reflexology for a better quality and longer night's sleep.

Tahira is very thankful that she had the opportunity to attend your workshop and could learn a routine of reflexology. This has made a huge improvement to the wellbeing of our family. We will make sure that reflexology is always a part of George's life.

When returning from school on Wednesdays after having reflexology George is generally in a happy mood. He will always show positive gestures and expression if we ask him about the session and mention your name.

Best regards

Tahira, Gary & George Crow.

Reflexology on the timetable during the school day, supported with the FRT framework, and the value of sharing skills with parents and carers empowers their lives.

> ## Tips for Reflexologists
>
> » Adapting techniques and working both feet together where possible. Feet need to feel secure and held through these movements. Bi-manual spine work was well received by George and very relaxing. You may need to adapt your position of delivery; do you ever stand up? I do.
> » Can a social story help preparation, communication, and ease anxiety beyond your touch?
> » The use of visual support must not be underestimated. It allows time for processing information and for language and can help with meaning. These supporting tools do not disappear like the spoken word.
> » Consider how you can also support the family.

Feedback from George

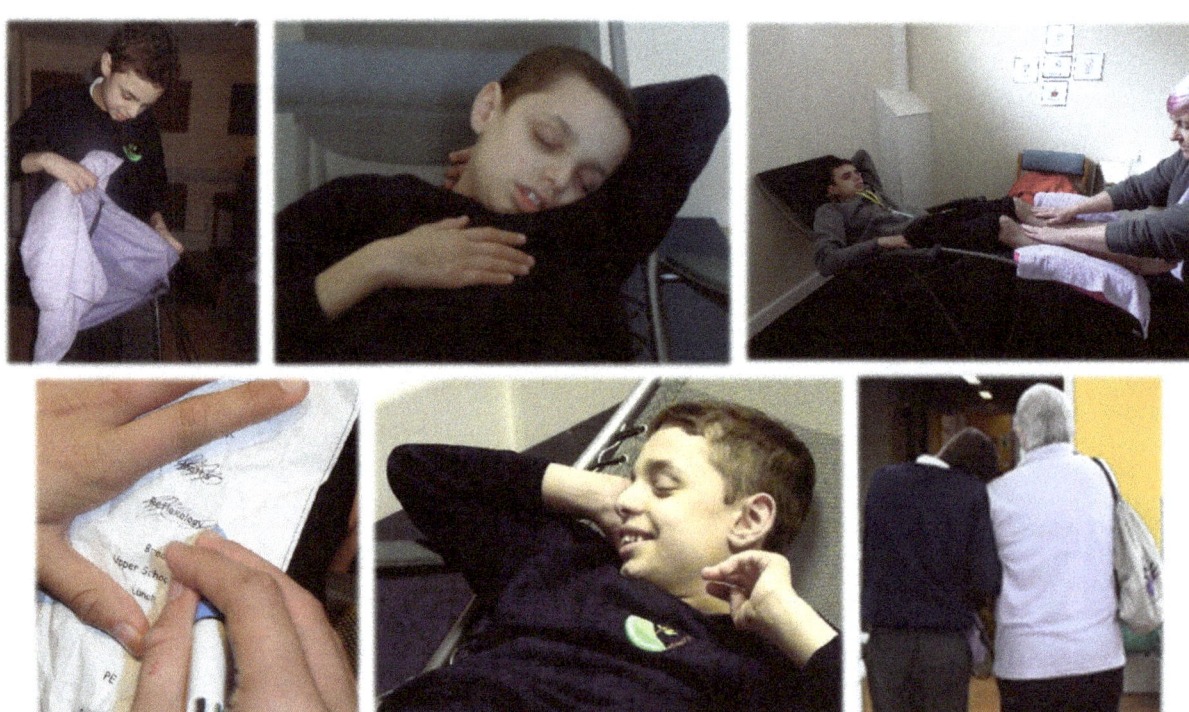

Gratitude and Learning

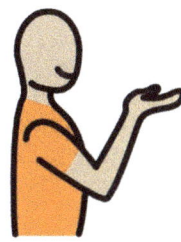

Thank You

Thank you, George, for accepting the invitation to come to the therapy room for reflexology. You have allowed me the opportunity to get to know you just a little bit and not just to work with you. You have helped me to become a better active listener and when I think back to our work together, I still see your smiles and hear your giggles and laughter at the end of the sessions. What wonderful evidence we have been able to share about our work together, the importance of providing a supportive environment, developing a good relationship, and how receiving the nurturing touch of reflexology can create such a meaningful connection.

Links and Further Information

Schwachman-Diamond Syndrome: www.sdsuk.org
National Autistic Society: www.autism.org.uk
Social Stories: www.carolgraysocialstories.com

Chapter 9: Meet Harry

'I give a big smile at the end of the session and help tidy up.'

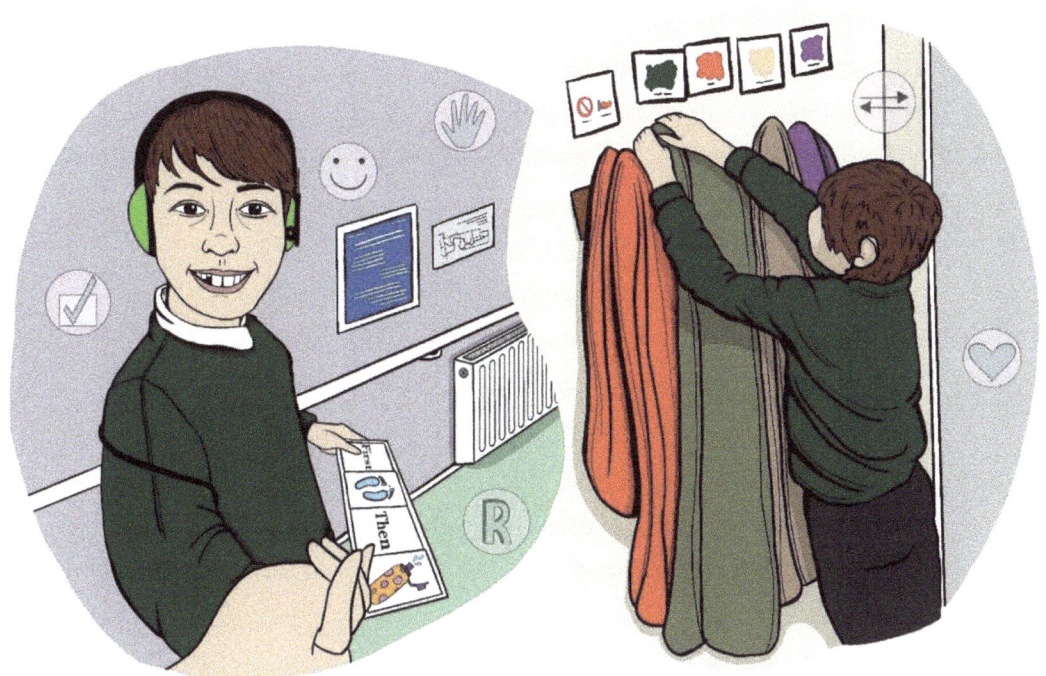

OUR WORK TOGETHER began in January 2020 just before Harry was nine years of age. (Who knew at that time in that year what the world had in store for us all!)

Fun loving, spirited, active, and a very fast young man. Fast in his activities, fast in moving on, fast with the time he could give his attention and focus to in the classroom.

Harry is autistic, he needs time to gather and process information and appropriate methods to help him with his communication, to bring him control and independence for some situations.

The Process

Teacher referral

The teacher said, 'There are occasions when the general workings and ongoing classroom activities can feel overwhelming for Harry and the noise around him will unsettle him. He can get easily distracted because of this and can quickly lose focus on tasks and activities.'

She continued, saying, 'At times Harry does find it very difficult to cope and to regulate his emotions. His responses may become unpredictable and sometimes his actions can be extremely distressing for him and to others around him. It is very important that we use meaningful methods of communication and allow time to support Harry.'

The teacher wanted him to:

- » experience time away from the busyness of the classroom;
- » be allowed time to process the information given by the therapist without interruption and time to feel and to respond to the touch;
- » to be offered choices in the therapy room, lights, music, blanket, etc.;
- » to begin to understand he could give his consent and to know he can ask to stop at any time;
- » to develop a relationship with a new member of staff who is offering something very different;
- » to take some responsibility for carrying the FRT toolkit and getting involved in using the contents, working with the therapist and following instructions to help set up the area;
- » accept the touch and show calmness and relaxation from receiving it;
- » indicate enjoyment of the session when returning to the classroom.

Classroom observation

I was able to take time to see Harry use his visual timetable. He studied the full timetable then took a symbol/picture/photo that was next in line and added it to his portable communication strip. This helped him to know what was going to happen now/first and then what was going to be happening next.

I listened carefully to the few words that staff used as instruction for him and the time they allowed for him to process the information.

Visual timetables

Visual timetables can be really useful as they are easily accessible, mobile, and a supportive way to help some children to understand the structure of the school day. They can be used at home, too. Some young people can become anxious if they do not know what is going to happen next and/or what activity they are moving on to.

Reducing the noise

You may notice Harry wearing some noise reduction earmuffs/ear defenders/noise cancelling headphones. These can help to reduce noise for any person whose hearing is sensitive to external noises, which could cause real discomfort and an unsettled response. When the sounds or noises are dulled or masked, it helps Harry to focus and to remain settled.

Sometimes he keeps them on in the therapy room. It does not matter. I do not insist he removes them, but on occasions he will remove them and pop them on the table or place them on his lap. If I were to insist on removal (why would I feel I needed to do that?), this would only raise levels of anxiety, which would not be very helpful for the intention of the session!

As the therapist, it is important that you create the best environment possible to help your young client feel safe, calm, and able to relax.

Communication and allowing time to process information

Some people find traditional forms of communication quite challenging; it can be difficult and confusing and so it is important to try to understand different methods that can offer support to help understanding and reduce stressful feelings.

At this time, Harry uses his 'first this and then …' communication strip. You'll see Harry and the communication strip on the story board.

Harry requires time to process information efficiently. It is important that he does not receive too much as this can overwhelm him and lead to frustration. He needs to be given time to make sense of the information. If it is provided in too much quantity and too quickly, it will not be meaningful.

There are many communication and sensory integration theorists. To me it is a fascinating subject and I would like to refer here to A. Jean Ayres, who was an occupational therapist, and educational psychologist and advocate for children with special needs in the USA. She became known for her work on sensory integration theory. Ayres talked about the process used by the brain to locate, sort, and make sense of all the information that was coming when trying to cope with and accomplish tasks. She described the challenges, which she terms 'sensory integrative dysfunction', as a sort of traffic jam in the brain. Some of the information would get through, some would get 'tied up in traffic' and certain parts of the brain would not get the sensory information needed in order to cope with what someone wants to do. This insight clearly helps me to work with young people with information processing difficulties; it reminds me to provide meaningful information, not too much, and allow sufficient time for it to go where it needs to go.

The principles of allowing time for the gathering and processing of information are the foundations on which the delivery of reflexology within the FRT framework is created.

Remind yourself that less of more = more.

Making choices

One of the personal learning targets for Harry for me to work towards during the session was to offer him a choice. He was working with this in class already, so it was great support that I could offer in my reflexology sessions. In the therapy session, I used the blankets for Harry to make choices. After it was clear that he liked using a blanket and that he understood, I began to introduce some different coloured blankets. Eventually we had four colours available as well as his choice not to use one at all. The interesting thing was that he didn't seem to have a favourite colour and he moved between them, a different one each week and sometimes none. Choosing and collecting and putting it back on the peg at the end of the session became part of his involvement in preparing for, finishing up, and tidying away, thus taking a little responsibility for the session.

Reflexology and reflection insights from my records
Before the touch

Harry needed time to prepare himself, changing the pictures on his communication strip, putting the toolkit on to his back, all helping with his preparation for transition from the classroom to the therapy room.

The walk to the therapy room is an important start to the therapy session; it gives me time to observe, listen, and helps me to decide on how he might be feeling. Was it a quick walk, was he unsettled, did he want to sign, did he smile, was he very quiet, did he look at his communication strip often for reassurance, etc.?

During the touch

Bringing in choices within the session, not just for the blankets, but perhaps encouraging Harry to indicate which movements he liked/preferred.

Harry was usually very keen to get going; once in the therapy room he wanted the touch! So, encouraging him to get involved was great, but it was done quite quickly. Depending on his frame of mind when he arrived, he would often say, let's get started!

Having fun! Harry loved singing so we made up a little song. We would sing it on the way and change the words occasionally in the therapy room, which brought some giggles, just a bit of fun. https://www.youtube.com/watch?v=xWOaO7Bfq6c

By session 9, 11th March, 2020, Harry seemed more comfortable with the routine of the session, but my records noted that on collection from the classroom, staff informed me he had been unsettled and fidgety. He had found being with others particularly difficult in the morning and seemed frustrated, exhibited behaviours that meant he had harmed himself and was very unsettled and they didn't know why. I wondered how he might settle with reflexology as they told me this. He did not take much time to look at his schedule, but turned for me to put the FRT toolkit on his back and we quickly walked side by side to the therapy room. He sat quickly, removed his shoes and socks and was ready. He was calm, he was still, he was silent and, importantly, so was I. We did not need to exchange any talk, my meaningful communication was through my touch, through my intention, and through my observation.

After the touch

Taking time to count down and finish, following instructions to pack away, show the next activity on the communication strip – it all seemed to be developing smoothly. We were getting to know each other, we had a regular slot on the timetable, the structure of the sessions worked well, and we were having some fun. I have to say I was very proud of the way the relationship was building and the value I could see that Harry and the class were beginning to derive from the sessions.

Note the date, March 2020! Little did we know that within the next two weeks the world was going to change, and a full COVID-19 lockdown would be enforced.

With stops and starts, in school, out of school, lockdowns, no lockdowns, the year disappeared and 2020 became an unsettled, unsure, 2021. If it was confusing and unsettling for us, how could we begin to help some of our young people understand what was going on. The answer was, generally, we couldn't!

On 18th May, 2021, Harry and I restarted our weekly sessions as life post-COVID seemed to be settling. On collection, I was informed he was unsettled, and it was suggested that a member of staff followed us down the corridor, reassurance for both Harry and me. He wanted to come along, he walked quickly straight to the therapy room and settled okay. He chose to hold on to the FRT toolkit and looked inside, lifting out the hand and the foot model. About ten minutes into the session, it was noted that he was suddenly unsettled and angry. This is where the video recording comes in very useful, as I can note down a time and a date and go back to look, listen, and reflect. I know I am repeating information here about the usefulness of the video, but it's worth it as it is such an important tool for my reflection.

Efficacy and effectiveness

Using the video recording, I get to hear my comments and see my actions and maybe this will help me work in a different way next time or to feel reassured that I did the best I could. On this occasion, it showed me Harry settled, but then suddenly sitting up and seemingly angry about something. He threw the foot model in my direction, which hit my arm. He kicked his feet at me and I sat back, to avoid contact.

'Harry', I said, 'when you threw the model it hit me, and it hurt my arm,' and I slowly rubbed the top of my left arm. I just felt I needed to tell him that his actions hurt me, and I quietly moved on. At no point did he remove his feet or attempt to get up. I continued with the touch.

The video showed that there was quietness in the therapy room for a few minutes and then Harry said 'Sorry.' I replied, 'Thank you Harry, I can see you are enjoying reflexology now.'

That is a big tear-jerker for me.

The challenges of sensory processing! I wonder what Harry was thinking about in those moments. Clearly something that overwhelmed him and he struggled to cope with whatever it was.

I did not take this personally; this was not against me. Think about the RECIPE if something like this happens during a session. It is crucial to use your skills and experience to calm and manage the situation.

Staff feedback

'Returning to the classroom, Harry would usually settle to an activity at his desk, he seemed calm and settled. I do really feel it was a positive helpful experience. He was always very keen to go with Lorraine.'

Parent feedback

Sharing a little video along with the feedback at the end of Harry's timetable sessions was really well received by his parents. They commented, 'It was so nice to see just a little bit of what happens in the therapy room, and we can tell that he is really relaxed.'

Feedback from Harry

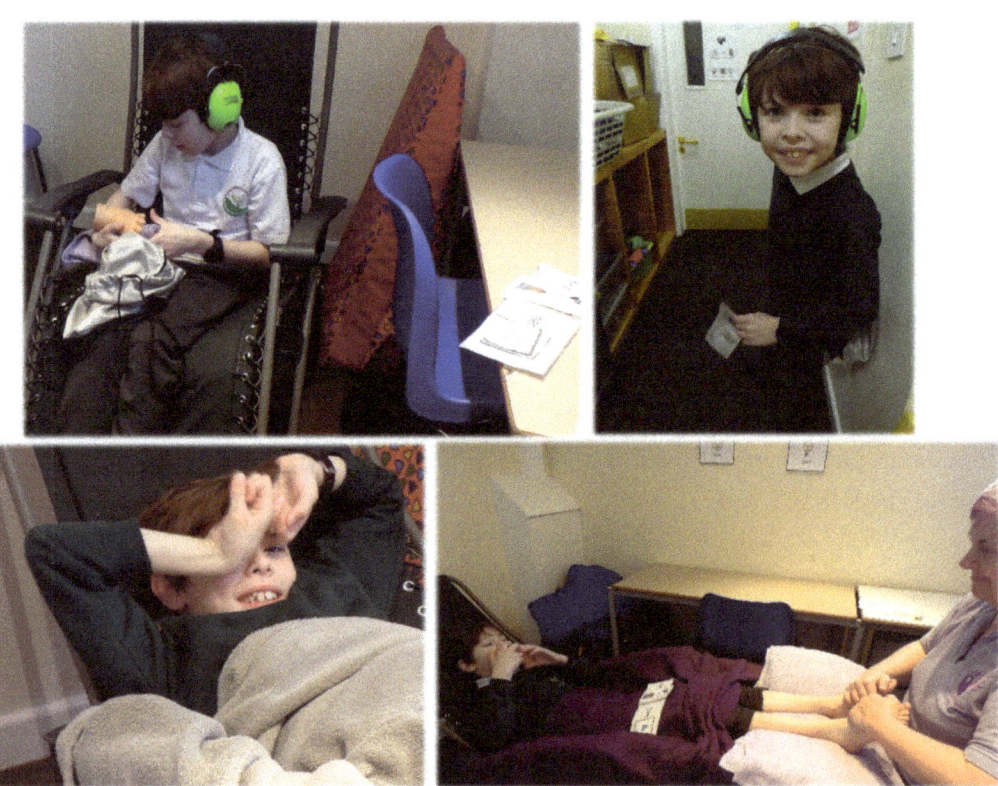

> ### Tips for Reflexologists
>
> » Consider a clear start and finish. I use a bi-manual thumb hold with the count-up to prepare, settle, and communicate the start, then repeat this hold with the countdown to finish to your session.
> » Using the video recorder and photos is reassurance and evidence collection for you, the therapist, and for the young person. It is a great tool for your learning. Parents sign the consent form to give permission for video and photos.
> » Regulate your voice. Know what is important to address. Avoid unnecessary actions that might lead to escalation of behaviour that is not acceptable or appropriate. Calm speaking voice, slow speaking, clear information – keep it short and meaningful.

Gratitude and Learning

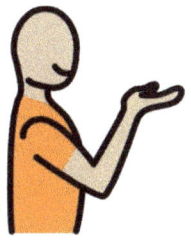

Thank You

Thank you, Harry, for accepting the invitation to come to the therapy room for reflexology. You have given me the opportunity to get to know you beyond the delivery of reflexology. You have helped me to become more aware of allowing sufficient time to process information. When I think about our sessions, 'Let's get started' always springs into my mind with a little singing.

Links and Further Information

National Autistic Society: www.autism.org.uk
Sensory Processing Difficulties: www.sensoryspectacle.co.uk

Chapter 10: Meet Scott

'Sometimes I stand up during the session and give Lorraine a big hug and a big smile.'

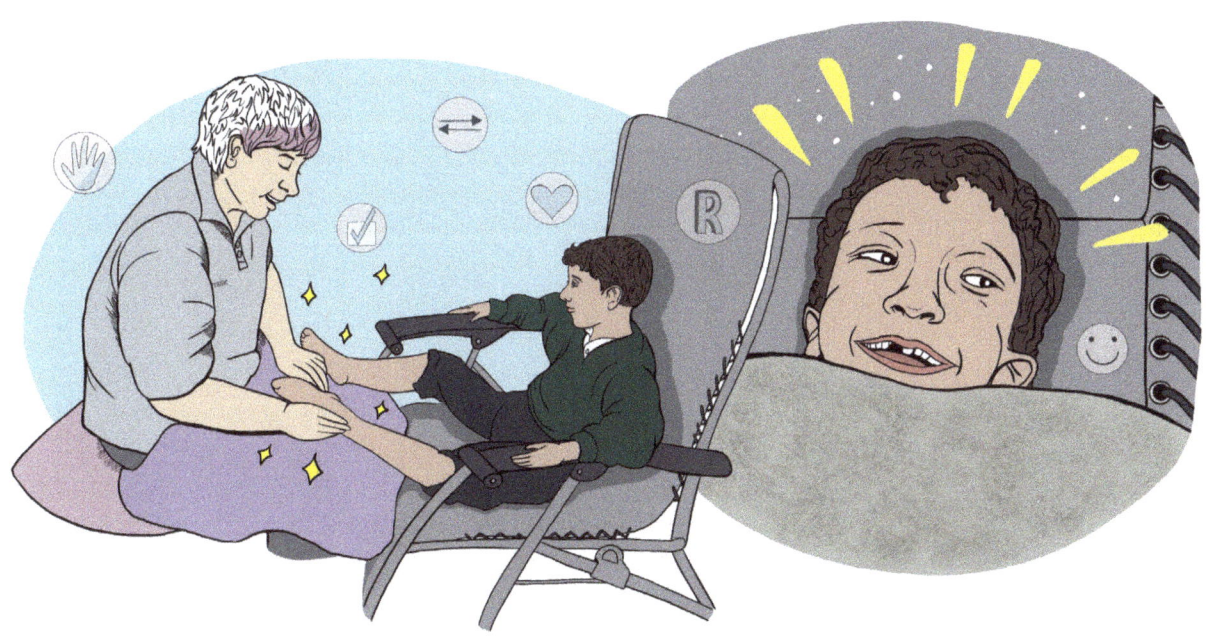

OUR WORK TOGETHER began in January 2013 when Scott was seven years of age. He was usually smiley and calm, which seems to denote a sense of happiness and contentment.

It changed significantly when it was therapy time, but not because he didn't enjoy the touch! Indeed, it changed significantly for any activity outside of the classroom. I was hopeful that the framework around the touch could help reduce his fretfulness and the session would meet the teacher referral expectations.

Scott is diagnosed with the rare genetic condition of cardio facial cutaneous (CFC) syndrome. He has global delay, severe visual and hearing impairment, and communication difficulties.

The Process

Teacher referral

The teacher noted on the referral that 'Scott found it very challenging to transition from the classroom to anywhere else within the school, which was quite understandable when you recognise the difficulties he was trying to work with.'

She went on to say, 'He can seem very anxious and unsettled if he is expected to change rooms, but he does however respond well to touch, encouragement, and likes to hold on to a person or on to objects.'

She was hopeful that the transition to the therapy room and to a new part of the school might help with his confidence in his ability to move to receive an activity that he enjoys.

The teacher wanted him to:

- » begin to feel more comfortable moving around the school;
- » develop a new relationship and become familiar and comfortable with a new member of staff;
- » develop an awareness of feet and lower leg, and she thought the session may help this;
- » recognise that he was in control of the session and give consent for the touch;
- » indicate enjoyment during the session.

Building confidence: classroom observation

Observation in class and discussion with staff helped me to understand that Scott had little or no hearing and had severe visual challenges. At times he found movement around the classroom difficult, which could be caused by changes in colours, light and dark, and/or floor type. I needed to think carefully about helping him to feel as reassured as possible on his transition from the classroom to the therapy room. Getting used to my voice and to the touch of me either holding his hand, or supporting his hand and forearm while walking alongside me. We played with the FRT toolkit bag so that he could feel the material of the bag and the towel. I found that this was helpful when moving along the corridor to the therapy room as it almost took his focus away from the difficulties and distractions that he seemed anxious about.

Before the touch

I greeted him clearly with his name so he knew I was talking to him and, importantly, I needed to crouch down and to be in front of him. Preparation included having good lighting and giving time to allow Scott to look towards me if he wanted to and to feel my hands. He often liked to feel my face as I was talking.

Scott had the opportunity to feel the FRT bag and I would guide his hand inside to feel the towel and find the pot of balm.

During the touch

Over the weeks of coming to the therapy room, Scott had the opportunity to sit in the large Lafuma chair and to experience the feel of the softer seat and what it felt like for him when I began to recline it.

Indicating enjoyment

Some weeks he placed his head gently on to the back of the seat and laughed as I slowly began to move it back into the recline position. I took this to be his permission to continue. In other weeks, as it began to tip back, he would move as if he wanted to sit up, so I took this as his decision to sit up for that session.

Interestingly, sometimes during the session he chose to shuffle forward and to stand up. The first time he did this I thought perhaps it was his way of saying 'I want to stop' *but*, to my surprise, he stood up, leant forward towards me, and gave me a big hug, then sat back down as if to say thanks, I'm liking this, please carry on. Well ... imagine how I felt. I'm getting a bit emotional just thinking about it now! Can you begin to imagine how you might feel? I don't need to imagine ... I know how you will feel!

For Scott this session was about allowing him the opportunity to make decisions, to carefully watch for subtle clues and cues. Body movements, reaching out of limbs, lifting of feet and legs, smiles, laughter, touch.

Sometimes Scott liked to hold a coloured light/torch. I would turn it on while it was still in the FRT toolkit, so he would feel and look for it. It stayed one colour and was not too bright, which meant he could safely hold it close to his face. Sometimes he would tap it on his cheek and then move it in front of his eyes. Other times, however, he would hold it for a short time and then either drop it on the floor or throw it! And our session would continue without it.

After the touch

We brought the reflexology session to an end with the recognisable squeeze and countdown. At the end of the countdown, the light was always switched off and Scott was encouraged to replace it in the FRT toolkit, which we would carry together as we returned to the classroom. We often had an empty crisp packet in the toolkit that acted as an object of reference, since Scott was usually returning to the classroom for snack time in the afternoon. Holding on to it on the way back signalled to Scott that he would have his snack when he returned to the classroom.

Reflexology and reflection insights from my records

Session 1, 16th January, 2013. We walked to the session with staff support. (I took his hand and supported under his arm. I was appreciative of the staff support; it was reassuring for both Scott and for me, and the member of staff came into the room.) Scott sat on the Lafuma chair. He was unsettled, a little fidgety and unsure of his surroundings, turning his head and looking around. I wondered what he could see. We played a bit with the music on and off, he held on to the FRT bag – he was not letting go! He allowed me to take his shoes off and hold his feet and he was sitting with the chair in the upright position. Total time in the therapy room, six minutes.

Session 2, 23rd January, 2013. Scott walked with assistance from a staff member, pausing midway along the corridor, hovering on his tip-toes, holding on to the member of staff for reassurance. He appeared unsettled by the flooring in the corridor at this point, where it changes to a darker covering. So, it was good to try to distract him a little. We scrunched the FRT toolkit and I got out the foot model. I'm not sure the model was too meaningful at this point, apart from the fact that he could hold it, chew it and it did give him a focus. The member of staff stopped by the door to the therapy room. Scott seemed okay to come in with me and session 2 went pretty much the same as session 1, but I recorded eight minutes in the therapy chair.

Session 3, 30th January, 2013. Scott walked without additional staff support! We held the FRT toolkit together, he came into the therapy room, sat down, and seemed quite settled. I removed his shoes and his socks; the chair was still upright. I wiped his feet and put some balm on. During the ten minutes (yes, ten minutes we had in the therapy room this time!), he stood up twice and gave me a hug!

By session 6, 27th February, 2013, Scott had begun to experience a slight reclining position while on the chair, but also was showing me that he didn't always want it reclined, as I mentioned previously. He did, however, always seem to be happy to have his shoes and socks removed. Together we had discovered his liking for being covered with a blanket so he could now make a choice, to have or not to have a blanket. We had also discovered that he liked the little red light and could feel for it in the toolkit. And he was enjoying weekly ten-minute sessions.

He was quite small in the Lafuma, so I added a soft pillow behind his back which seemed to help him to settle. He just looked more comfortable.

Some nice sounds and vocalisations today –I don't remember hearing those before – and a giggle. I looked back at the video but couldn't truly establish a particular movement; however, he was very happy. He just enjoyed the whole experience.

Session 14, 24th April, 2013. Shoes and socks off, chair reclined, loving the blanket, very smiley, sat up and gave me a hug! Returned to the chair and happy for the touch of reflexology to continue. Twelve minutes of touch time on his feet and then, when he sat up, he crossed his legs and held out his hands. I couldn't resist a count up and a few minutes of repetition on his fingertips and sweeping along his forearms, but it's still important to count down to know it is coming to the end. In total we had 15 minutes in the therapy room today!

I wrote, 'Cheeky Scott! Had enough of my feet, here are my hands!'

By the session recorded on *15th March, 2013*, most weeks he was choosing to have the chair reclined. Today, however he was full of cold and quite congested. Still wanting to come along to the therapy room, he walked well with me to the therapy room and he did not want the chair reclined. Totally understandable, and great that he made the choice. A longer session than usual; I think he was tired and was just accepting the touch. In total, 20 minutes of touch time.

Session 17 at 20 minutes was a one-off! Most of the final five sessions were recorded at 14 minutes of touch time.

12th June, 2013 was our final session together. The chair was fully reclined, the blanket was over his head and he received 14 minutes touch time. He has really got used to the session and is enjoying the touch.

Most weeks he chose the green blanket, sometimes the red, but never the beige or the purple. I don't think it was necessarily the colour he could see, I feel it was more likely the difference in the feel and texture of the blanket that meant he was drawn to the green one as it was much thicker and had some weight to it.

Although this was not an official weighted blanket, I think it offered a similar feeling of security. Weighted blankets, gilets, shoulder covers, gloves, are all objects that can sometimes help the body to feel calm, to feel settled and reassured. The green blanket was often a favourite in the therapy room, and I do think its thickness and weight was more likely to be the reason than the colour of it. I would recommend you try a weighted one. The makers of these blankets often recommend them for sleeping but they can be used in many settings. They are also referred to as therapeutic blankets; the pressure replicates the experience of being held or hugged to relax the nervous system, calming and reducing rapid heart rates.

Teacher feedback

'Due to his visual challenges, Scott understandably finds it very challenging to explore the spaces around him and takes a while to feel comfortable with new people.

'The staff team have commented how well he has accepted Lorraine and seems to have become familiar and happy with the touch therapy of reflexology.

'I feel that the approach Lorraine has used is similar to our classroom support, with the toolkit acting as an object of reference. As soon as it is felt in the classroom it has helped him to get involved and perhaps to recognise where he is going and what is going to be happening. Lorraine would bring the iPod and music along as part of the toolkit, the music was the same each week and different to anything we used for sessions in class, and she would rub a little balm on to the back of his hand, which I feel helped him to recognise and prepare for the session.'

Feedback from Scott

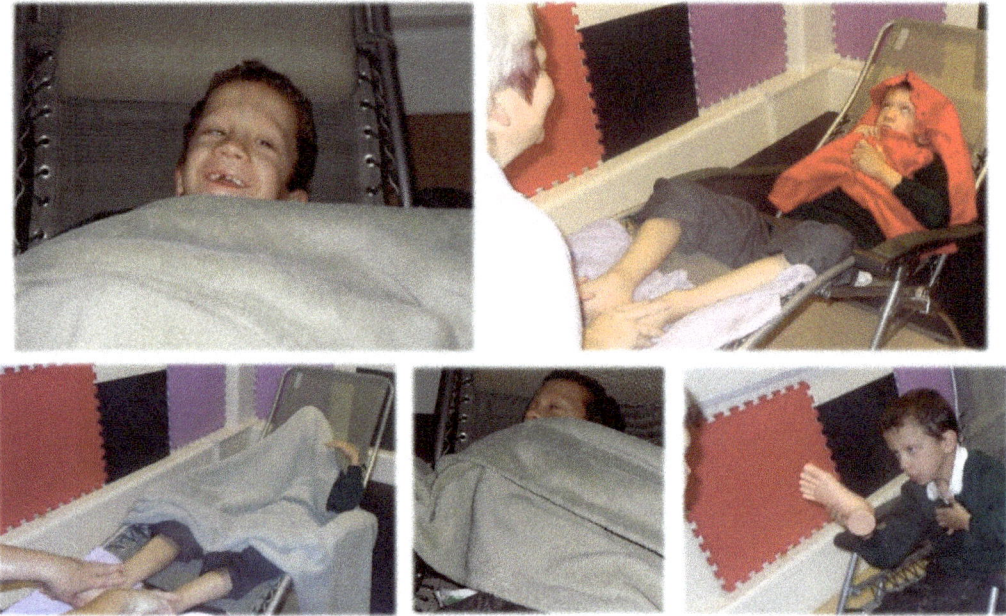

Tips for Reflexologists

» Requests to stop the touch do not always mean a request to stop the session completely. A hug from Scott taught me that!
» Repetition of movement creates familiarity and reassurance. If there is a favourite or a preferred movement/technique, repeat it and repeat it, think about the intention of your session within this setting.
» Use of touch, object, and calm voice used close to the ear to guide and encourage.

Gratitude and Learning

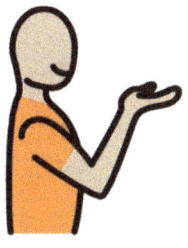

Thank You

Thank you, Scott, for accepting the invitation to come to the therapy room for reflexology. You have allowed me the opportunity to get to know you just a little bit and not just to work with you. You have reminded me that thanks can be shown in many different ways and you remind me every session of the value that a repetition of your favourite techniques can bring to your calmness and enjoyment of the session.

Links and Further Information

Cardiofaciocutaneous Syndrome: www.cfcsyndrome.org
Mencap: www.mencap.org.uk/learning-disability-explained/conditions/global-development-delay

Chapter 11: Meet Oliver

'Just because I remove my feet, it doesn't mean I am not enjoying reflexology. Just give me a few moments ... They'll be back.'

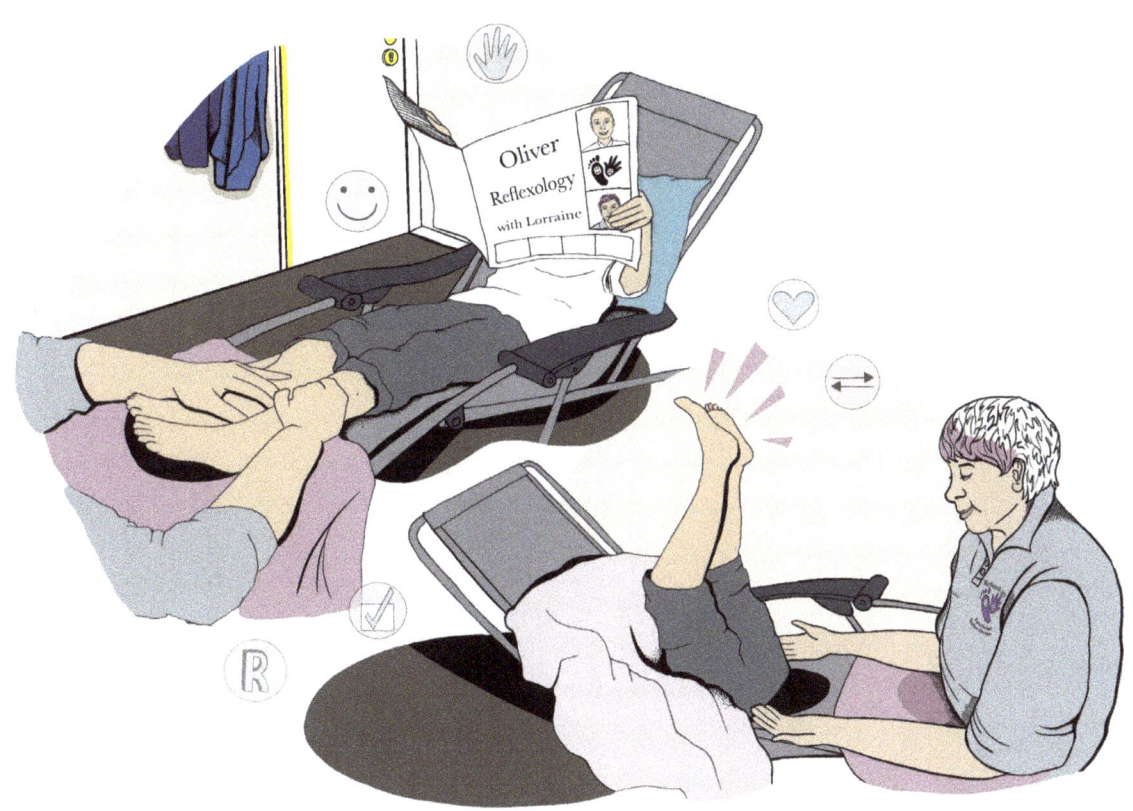

OUR WORK TOGETHER began in 2016 when Oliver was ten years of age. He has a special interest, loving a newspaper. Creating one with him for his reflexology session was super supportive for him and very interesting for me. It seemed to provide him with a comforting space. He couldn't see me but enjoyed the opportunity to turn the pages and see some pictures of himself in the therapy room and some pictures of the movements. I could ask him which one he was looking at and if he wanted to feel the movement, a valuable addition to the toolkit to meet Oliver's needs and for us to make a connection.

Oliver is diagnosed with ASD, ADHD, with associated difficulties with communication, and, referring to my records from 2016, he was taking part in a sleep study as at that time his sleep pattern was very irregular. He was taking some medication at home which helped with his anxiety and used an asthma inhaler.

The Process

Teacher referral

The teacher referral shared that Oliver generally had a very short attention span which they were working with, offering space, movement, and time away from activities. He often looked for attention and constant reassurance and on occasions he would get very angry, sometimes aggressive.

The teacher went on to say that she noticed a frustration in many activities during the day. He may display a lack of interest, but that they are aware he has a very unsettled sleep pattern, which could have an impact on how he is able to cope during the day with demands or requests from staff and from his peers, and on his ability to learn.

He worries about leaving the classroom, can get quite anxious if the whole class is not together, and constantly asks about what he might be missing, which means he finds it difficult to focus and cope with the activity they would like him to take part in or the job he may have been asked to do.

The teacher wanted him to:

- » experience time away from the busyness of the classroom and to accept and cope with the fact that it is okay to take time away from the classroom;
- » try to settle himself and regulate how he is feeling in the therapy room;
- » be encouraged and given an opportunity to talk about how he is feeling or use pictures of emotions;
- » indicate enjoyment (or not) of the session when returning to the classroom;
- » use the session and reflexology to support his well-being, which perhaps may influence his sleep pattern.

Classroom observation

Oliver was keen to please his teacher, but always seems to be wanting to move on to the next activity (unless he is using Lego, which seems currently to be his favourite activity). I noticed that Oliver is often asking if things are okay, and what to do next. He was constantly looking for the teacher's attention and was showing a general anxiousness even during the short time that I was able to observe, finding it difficult to settle and focus for more than a few minutes.

A short note on the efficacy

So much happened throughout these sessions during the time that I was privileged to support Oliver that it is difficult to condense it into a short story. But I know you will love the points; I think they are worth sharing. I just can't fit them all in, but I'll try my best. So much more than 'just the touch', and 'what very interesting teacher feedback'.

Building a Relationship and Lifting Self-esteem

Before the touch

Oliver could see that reflexology was on his timetable. He found transition away from the classroom difficult, especially if he was going without the rest of the class, but it was important for him to know that this would be happening.

When I arrived to collect him, staff would reassure him that he would continue with the same work when he returned to class so he would not miss anything.

Reflexology and reflection insights from my records

As shown in the illustration at the head of the chapter, Oliver is holding a newspaper. Yes, it was a real newspaper and at the time he enjoyed looking through the pages and liked to take it around with him. So, I designed a reflexology newspaper that he could bring along to the therapy room. This helped him to feel a little calmer and, knowing it was something he felt he needed, it helped him to prepare for the session and transition with a little more ease, along with happily carrying the FRT toolkit on his back.

During the touch

In our first session, on 13th September, 2016, Oliver was happy to follow instructions to remove shoes and socks and, interesting for me, it revealed a few verrucae. He was happy for me to touch and work with his feet (he was behind the newspaper). I worked carefully around and closely to the verrucae; he did not show any signs of discomfort. *(Here, it is important to know and remember your responsibilities as a reflexologist and know your boundaries, working as part of the multidisciplinary team. See where I took this information in the reflexology reflection and top tips.)*

I didn't see much of Oliver for the first few weeks as he was behind his paper. I also put into the paper some photos of a few of the techniques I was using and referred, for example, to the photo on page one or page five when I used that specific movement, and he enjoyed finding them.

Each week I offered a blanket, but for the first few weeks the newspaper was his priority. It was important here for him to become familiar not only with me but also the structure and timing of the therapy session and, most of all, to realise that he had a choice in the therapy room.

Session 6, 18th October, 2016. Oliver put the newspaper on the table and said 'I think I would like the red blanket today.'

This was also an interesting session; the blanket was over his head, which, of course, is absolutely fine. We do not need to see faces to recognise when relaxation is happening. And being under the blanket or pulling a jumper up over a face, as you will see in other studies, is often a reassuring comfort.

Allowing time for self-regulation

During the early sessions Oliver would occasionally lift his legs right up into the air. What I learned from this was the importance of allowing him time. I needed to be a little patient and not insist that he replace his legs but wait until he did and offered his feet to indicate his readiness for me to continue. It was clear that he was enjoying it, by the fact that he replaced his feet, but that he needed a little extra time to regulate and time to prepare for more.

The length of his touch time was increasing and, in this session, he was settled for 14 minutes. At this point he said, 'I think I am missing choosing time', and I asked him if he would like to stop reflexology. After a countdown and a quick sort out to put the towel in the bag, he popped the toolkit on his back, and we had a very quick walk to return to the classroom. I said thank you and that I would see him next week. 'Okay' was the reply.

The following week I recorded something very different after the touch.

After the touch

Session 7, 1st November, 2016. After 15 minutes of touch time, he walked slowly side by side with me to the classroom. We met a lady who was on a tour visiting the school who stopped to say hello. He was seeking for my hand. I held it reassuringly and together we greeted the visitor, and he told her 'Lorraine gave me reflexology.' No wonder I documented how delighted I was. Not only that he found reassurance by holding my hand, so I had become a familiar person, but also what a great result it was to speak to the visitor and refer to me and reflexology.

Session 9, 15th November, 2016 is worth a mention as Oliver was settled enough to allow a new person to be in the therapy room. Although they were sitting out of sight, he knew they were there and they were doing some filming as I began to make a wonderful video for a presentation that I was preparing to share in Taiwan in 2017.

I had prepared Oliver the week before, with a photograph of the gentleman who was coming into the session and his name, which I do think helped with his preparation, as he knew what was going to be happening. As we started the session, video on, socks and shoes off, chair reclined, I began to wipe Oliver's feet. He popped his hands behind his head, took in a large breath and let out a beautiful aaaahhhhhhhh on the out breath. No one can tell me that he was not enjoying this opportunity!

I took some photos of the underside of Oliver's feet to share with the school nurse. It was not my responsibility to diagnose a verruca. If we had not had a school nurse, I would have recommended the parents to check with the pharmacist or GP, but we used this as an opportunity to send a little information home to the whole school about foot health.

A verruca could cause discomfort in some children, even to the point of them being unsettled and in pain when walking, or even just wearing shoes.

Session 13, 20th December, 2016. I had music playing in the room on arrival and Oliver asked me to turn it off. This presented no problem and it was very important for him to exercise choice! I respected his choice, but on this day, I had a new CD playing quietly, awaiting his usual instruction. He said, and I wrote, 'Oh that's nice music.' I asked him if he would like it left on. 'Yes' was his reply.

By session 17, 7th February, 2017, Oliver had begun to tell me some of the movements he liked. He was not able to tell me why he liked them, but he just had a preference, which was great because I could add more repetitions of those into the session. He particularly liked the work on his toes.

It didn't all go to plan and continue to improve at such a beautifully smooth rate. He often asked, 'What am I missing in the classroom?' I made a note of this in session 19.

Efficacy and effectiveness

What I observed throughout the sessions was Oliver's increased acceptance of leaving the classroom. He was coping much better, managing to remain calm. I don't think he was masking because he engaged and got involved with making decisions and making choices, but he also had the choice to stop and he did know this. The touch time increased. I think it was a real boost to his confidence.

I did not receive feedback from home about any improvement in sleep, but I am pleased with the outcome of the sessions and how they developed during the school day, and with the teacher feedback.

Teacher feedback

After many weeks, staff commented on noticing a difference as Oliver returned from reflexology. The teacher said, 'He seemed to be enjoying the session as he had occasionally volunteered a little information about the big chair and having his feet rubbed and he does not seem quite so uptight about leaving the room.'

The teacher went on to say that she thought the outcome of the sessions was positive and was a result of the whole framework that the classroom team and I had implemented.

Feedback from Oliver

L: Have you enjoyed coming for reflexology every week?

O: Sometimes.

L: What did you like about reflexology?

O: The big chair (I would have liked him to answer the movements on his feet but okay, the chair was a new experience and perhaps encouraged him to relax 'beyond the touch').

L: Was there one movement that you really liked?

O: Pressing my toes. I liked pressing on my toes a lot. I like my big toes together. I liked the sweep up the leg, you do that lots.

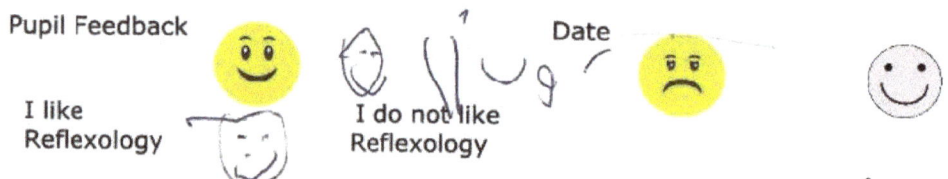

I am reassured by the facts that at no point did he refuse to come along to the therapy room, the touch time increased to a full 20 minutes, he made some choices, and his anxiousness about leaving the classroom was reduced. He never did miss choosing time, as the teacher made sure this activity was available for him on his return.

Further Feedback from Oliver

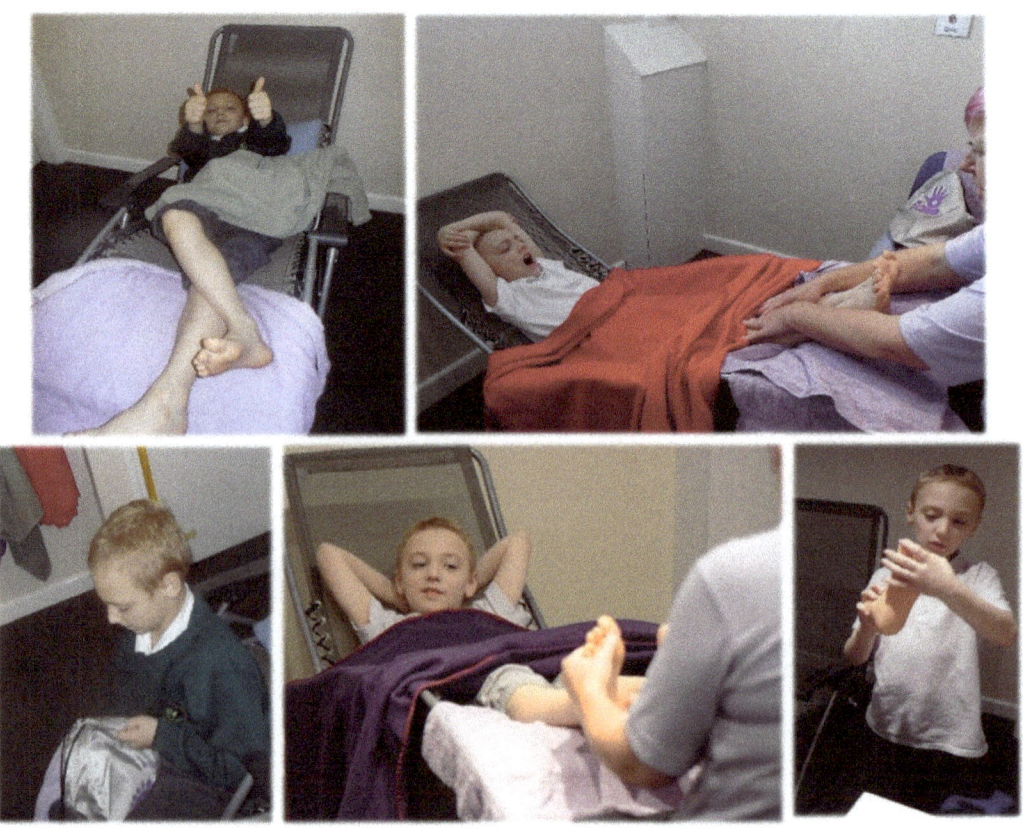

Tips for Reflexologists

» Don't be too quick to dismiss removal of feet or hands as not liking the movement. Allow time for that young person to regulate and decide if touch can continue.
» Don't assume that just because your client asks you to turn the music off that they will never want it. Perhaps it's the kind of music you are offering, perhaps it's just the mood of the moment.
» Where possible, ascertain a favourite technique that you can repeat throughout your reflexology sessions. Remember the intention for this session.

Gratitude and Learning

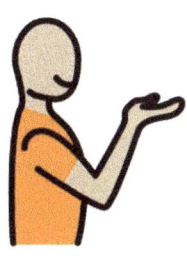

Thank You

Thank you, Oliver, for accepting the invitation to come to the therapy room for reflexology. You have allowed me the opportunity to get to know you just a little bit and not just to work with you. Working with you has taught me to appreciate the importance of time for self-regulation.

Links and Further Information

National Autistic Society: www.autism.org.uk
ADHD (Attention deficit hyperactivity disorder): www.Nhs.Uk/Conditions/Attention-Deficit-Hyperactivity-Disorder-Adhd/

Chapter 12: Meet Harley

'My favourite place is under the blanket, sometimes I pull it down a little and take a look at my feet and a look at Lorraine.'

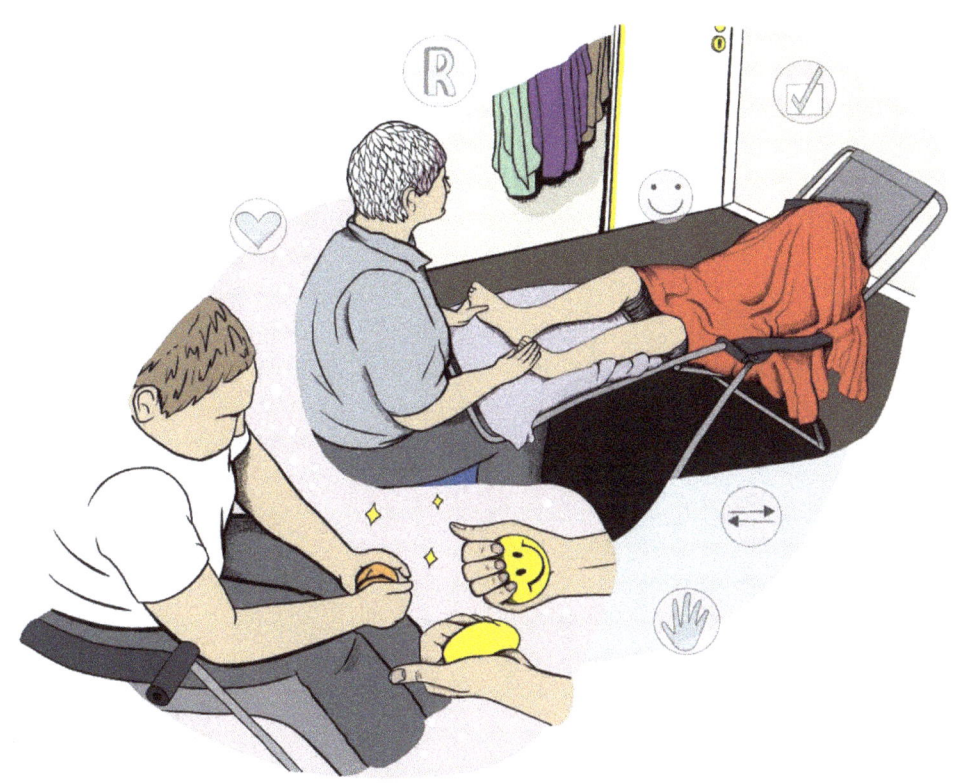

OUR WORK TOGETHER begins in October 2016 when Harley was 12 years of age.

He was sometimes very quiet, sometimes very loud, sometimes exhibiting short bursts of energy, but often subdued and lethargic, giving the appearance of being downbeat, sometimes almost sad.

Harley had difficulties with language, learning, attention, motor skills and self-help skills. He has a diagnosis of epilepsy. He can sometimes experience blepharitis, which may cause irritation and discomfort.

Here I am, six years on and reflecting on my records, recognising that I have been learning 'big time' from the young people I supported (and continue to support) and Harley was an important participant in that learning.

I talked to Harley about my reason for wanting to write a book so that other young people could read a little about reflexology and about his experience in the therapy room and headteachers might like to offer it in their schools when they hear what he has to say.

As he shrugged his shoulders and gave a little smile, he replied, 'Mmmm yep, it's okay. I quite liked reflexology.' So, together, we have decided what information might be helpful for you.

The Process

Teacher referral

At the time of the referral, the teacher wrote, 'Harley was often very easily distracted and needed a lot of support throughout the day to remain engaged. Sometimes he displayed very loud and distracting behaviours, which not only unsettled him but also has an impact, distracting and unsettling his friends and peers.'

The notes I referred to that I made during my meeting with the teacher and classroom staff read that at times Harley can struggle to regulate and control his emotions, leading to difficulty settling himself. Harley's self-esteem is low and he often looks and seems sad. They mentioned he was having difficulty sleeping, his pattern was unsettled, so felt it was not surprising that he is usually tired and easily distracted during the school day.

The teacher asked: Could the support from reflexology therapy, receiving this caring touch, encourage Harley to feel a little more relaxed? Could it help him with his sleep, which might help him to feel better during the day?

Naturally, as reflexologists reading this will know, I couldn't give her a definite answer to this question. My suggestion was more along the lines of: if his sleep pattern improves, he may feel better during the day, though any improvement might not be due to the reflexology as various other factors could influence this.

Emotional resilience

The teacher wanted him to:

» experience 1:1 time away from the busyness of the classroom;
» be introduced to a different type of support through the positive touch of reflexology therapy;

» experience a quiet environment, feeling safe and calm to express feelings and generally talk about anything he might want to;
» express in some way an enjoyment (or not) of the session when returning to the classroom.

Classroom observation

I was able to make two observations at different times to join in activities in the classroom, which was helpful. Harley very rarely lifted his head up; he avoided catching the eye of the teacher. I could see he would occasionally glance sideways and follow her movements around the room. If he was asked anything directly, he shrugged his shoulders and sighed. I could tell the teacher was trying to give him the confidence to show he could answer by asking questions he knew the answer to. However, he would rather avoid saying anything.

Reflexology and reflection insights from my records
Preparation and the invitation

I referred to the corridor display about reflexology that Harley passed every day in school. There were some pictures of his friends. The photos, symbols, and wording that went along with these referred to reflexology being calming and helping people to relax and feel good.

Having a choice

Harley was invited to visit the therapy room to have a look around. I showed him how the Lafuma chair worked, and he had a try as it reclined. He noticed the blankets hanging up. I asked him if he had a favourite colour as he would be able to choose if he would like to use one.

I think this was useful and helpful for Harley. I talked about reflexology, such as what happens when he gets ready for reflexology, including removing his shoes, socks, and cleaning and creaming, and the touch to his feet.

It's important to note here that Harley did not need to use the FRT toolkit as an object of reference, but I thought I would carry it when I went to the classroom as he might carry it, feeling he was getting involved in some way.

Sessions 1-3, 4th October, 2016-18th October, 2016. When I arrived at the classroom, each time he took a deep breath, gave a bit of a huff/sigh, as if he was saying 'Okay, I'll come but it's a bit of an effort.' I also wondered whether he was embarrassed in front of his friends. I was aware, too, that it might mean 'Do I have to come?' He did have the choice and I made sure he knew that each time, so it was interesting that I received this reaction, but each time he came. Possibly this was just his way of letting me know that it was his choice, and making sure that others in the class were aware that it was his choice. This is why I like to refer to my sessions as an invitation to the therapy room. As much as the initial consent and permission for the session is signed for by the parent, it is entirely the choice of the young person to decide to come along and to continue, or to stop the sessions at any time. Consent and ongoing consent are essential.

During the touch

From the classroom, in sessions 1–3, his body language was interesting. He would shuffle along the corridor and I would describe his shoulders as rounded, his head lowered, and gaze looking down. I tried to encourage a little engagement and interaction. It went along the lines of, 'It's nice to see you today, your work looked good in the classroom. What were you finishing?' etc., but he chose not to engage in the early weeks.

He would choose a blanket, usually the red one and be underneath it from start to finish. (And that is absolutely fine: he was in the therapy room, he had removed shoes and socks, he had offered his feet and at no point were they removed. I didn't need to see his face.)

Session 4, 1st November, 2016, following the half term break. In this session there was a little breakthrough via the toolkit. Harley took the bag from me in the classroom, for the first time. He pushed his water bottle in through the gathered top and then threw the straps over his shoulder for a short time before bringing it down as we walked along the corridor and swinging it from side to side. It only had a towel inside, but that didn't matter. I bet you can imagine the inner smile from me as he decided to get involved. Such a big moment, yet one might think it merely a tiny step.

Session 5, 15th November, 2016. I was aware that his upright feet had gently dropped outwards and the tension throughout and around his ankles had softened. He initiated a little conversation. I made a note of it as it was something very new to the session.

H: 'I've not had a very good week.'

L: 'Well, I am really pleased to see you and really pleased you chose to come along for reflexology today, thank you for that' and continued with 'Would you like to tell me about your week?'

Quite a long silence ensued – well over a minute; I didn't interrupt his thoughts. I wanted to hear but I didn't just want to be the empathetic listener. Deep down I was hopeful he might share and that we might start a conversation.

H: 'Not really.' (Well, that told me!)

L: 'I'm here to listen if there is ever anything, not just now, but anytime if you would like to pop in, you know where my room is.'

H: No reply.

Did it matter? Absolutely not. He wanted to come along, and accepted the invitation for reflexology, he initiated conversation to tell me things were difficult and, most important of all, he settled and offered his feet.

At this point I was still hopeful he might chat a little more during the session, but he didn't.

Session 11, 20th December, 2016. My records note end of term tiredness is evident throughout the school. Harley seemed quite keen to come along and he led the way.

9–10 minutes into the session, Harley suddenly tensed. He opened his eyes quite wide, looking up towards the ceiling and uttering some unusual sounds. I do remember this moment quite well. I spoke to him but he did not acknowledge me with either a look or a shrug of the shoulders, which was his more usual response. I felt a little bemused and also felt that it seemed as if it took minutes of my time, but it probably was more like a few seconds, before I recognised that he was having a seizure.

So, what to do? Reassure, as you do not know how much a person is hearing. Importantly, know the protocol for that young person and what is required within the environment you are working.

NB: To the best of my knowledge, there is no existing evidence suggesting that receiving reflexology will trigger a seizure. Awareness has come a long way since I first started my training in reflexology. The Epilepsy Society now actively supports and talks positively about complementary therapies, as often those individuals experiencing seizures may live with elevated levels of worry, apprehension, and anxiety.

To complete session 11, my notes document that he sat quietly, chair in upright position. Needed to use the toilet and was offered the option to come back to the quiet therapy room. He did, and took his water out of the FRT bag. Class teacher informed; seizure noted on class records.

Session 20, 21st March, 2017. Completing the 20 sessions and finishing for the Easter break, we shared relaxing therapy time and sometimes a little chat. In answer to my question,

L: 'How are you feeling about coming along each week?'

H: A quick shrug of his shoulders, and a stillness and quietness in the room. I waited …'I quite like it.' Oh yes … that will do for me! Thank you, Harley.

In the last few weeks, before returning to the classroom, I introduced some breathing and self-care hand reflexology techniques; he rather liked the fun of the squeezy balls. There is good reason for introducing them other than bringing a bit of fun, which is always a nice way to finish. We know, as reflexologists, the effect of pressure and coverage over the solar plexus area and the many benefits of breathing techniques alongside the squeeze.

Efficacy and effectiveness

There was a real difference noted in his positivity when coming along for sessions, as well as during the sessions with the relaxation and position of his feet.

He would still choose the red blanket but, in later sessions, snuggled it under his chin, left his face uncovered and closed his eyes. This suggested to me that he was feeling comfortable within the space of the therapy room and comfortable throughout the session to close his eyes and not feel awkward about doing this in front of me. It was almost as if he had given himself permission and allowed himself to say it is okay to relax.

I would like to think that the reflexology therapy room and framework that supported the session helped to introduce Harley to a new touch therapy experience, and even if at that time he was not able to recognise the impact and the effect it was having on his inner calmness, it might be something he can return to at a future date, knowing he enjoyed the sessions.

He particularly liked the effleurage that was included on his lower leg. The method of the delivery of my reflexology includes using a repetitive, rhythmical effleurage link between the reflexology techniques, knowing the many benefits of using this movement along the non-glabrous skin. I could feel, see, and hear the responses. Relaxation and softening of the calf muscles, softening of the ankle rigidity, feet dropping outwards, snuggling under the blanket, closing of the eyes. Alongside the initial shallow breathing that began to deepen, there was a stillness and a real sense of calmness 'in the moment'.

The long-term aim would be to encourage him to have a regular session as part of his lifestyle. It may not be just the touch of reflexology, but a combination of other therapies that may be able to support Harley in the future.

As reflexologists will know, using the squeezy balls provides additional support because they cover the solar plexus area and we can calm with additional counting up, squeezing and breathing, repeating, etc. This fits nicely into my sessions; we count up and then count down.

Harley took some of the balls back to the classroom ☺ and was occasionally encouraged to squeeze, to count, to breathe. I do know he used them for a short time, encouraged by his teacher.

Part of my role, as a reflexology therapist and a member of the multidisciplinary team, is to feed back at regular intervals to staff and parents, and at the end of the sessions to provide a short report about the values, responses, how the sessions have progressed, and some photos. Harley was able to be involved with that process of making a paper copy which, at that time, was filed in class and sent home.

Pupil Feedback Harley Date 21.3.17

I like Reflexology   I do not like Reflexology

This serves at least two purposes.

1. It helps to bring, as clearly as possible, an end to his sessions. They are finished because they have come to the end of the number allocated and not for any other reason.

2. It involves the pupil in giving their feedback – giving them a voice is so important.

Teacher feedback

'We generally don't often see Harley looking happy, but he usually returns from the reflexology sessions with a smile and settles quietly into his work; it might be helping that, at the moment on his timetable, he returns to a lesson that he likes.

'When I asked Harley if he enjoys reflexology, Harley said, "It's all right", and then "I quite like it".

'I said that was good to hear and then asked, what do you like about it? A shrug of the shoulders!

'I wanted to remind him, you know you have a choice each week. You can choose to go along with Lorraine. "I'll probably go".

'I would say he just looks brighter and relaxed on his return. His mood is brighter.'

Feedback from Harley

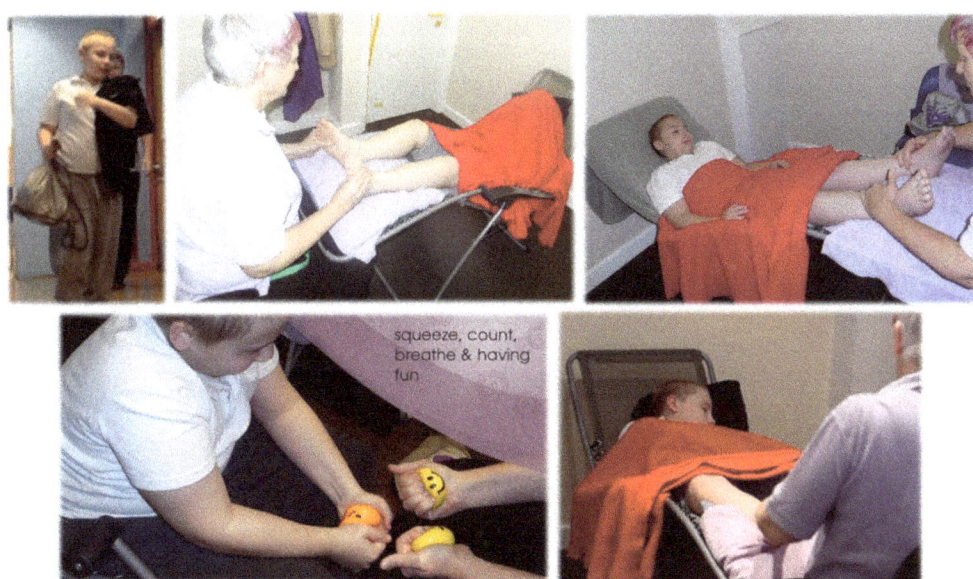

Tips for Reflexologists

» Know the protocols in place should a medical situation arise.
» Offer choices; this will help them to feel involved in the session and may encourage interaction, but just allow it to develop at its own pace.
» Record and document the smallest details and points as they arrive. Collect all your evidence to recognise how your sessions support emotional resilience.

Gratitude and Learning

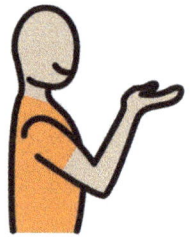

Thank You

Thank you, Harley. By accepting the invitation to join me in the therapy room for reflexology, you have provided me with the chance to get to know you a little bit better. You helped me to recognise I can gather valuable evidence to show the many benefits of our time together by observing the changes in your body language and listening to the sounds of your shoe shuffle and footsteps before and after the session.

Links and Further Information

Epilepsy: www.epilepsysociety.org.uk
Blepharitis, eye conditions: www.nhs.uk/conditions/blepharitis
Generalised Anxiety Disorder GAD: www.nhsinform.scot > illnesses-and-conditions

Chapter 13: Meet Cedric

'I love the sweeping movement up my lower leg, and sometimes I settle back and get comfy in the big chair.'

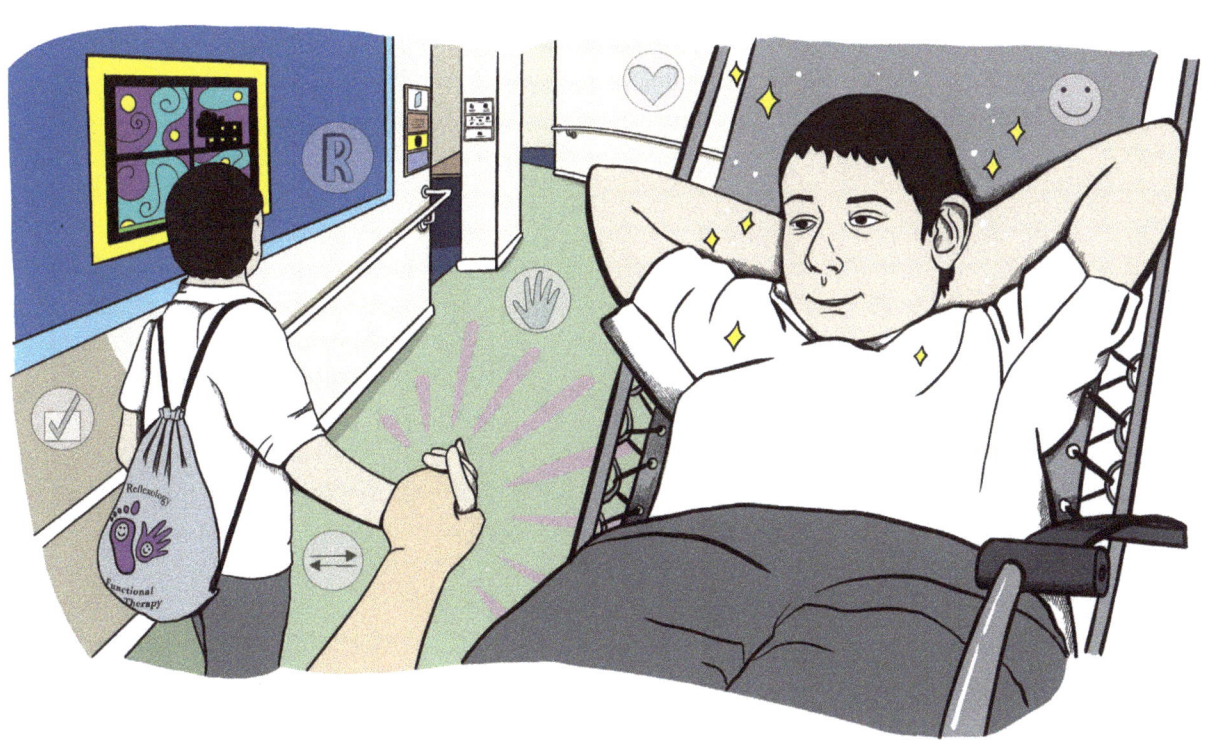

OUR WORK TOGETHER began in February 2019 when Cedric was eight years of age.

He is very lively, a little bustling in his actions in the classroom, wanting things to happen straight away and finding it challenging to wait once he has an idea of what he wants to happen.

Cedric is autistic with global delay, intellectual difficulties, and severe communication difficulties.

The Process

Teacher referral

Based on the teacher's referral, I noted that Cedric requires regular sensory breaks which may involve him moving around the classroom, taking some time in an alternative space and/or some deep pressure and stillness. He has a short attention span, which classroom staff try to work with, but he is very easily distracted and does seek a lot of attention. The teacher mentioned that he can seem distressed because he gets frustrated and will often cry, but is not able to express why.

The teacher said that Cedric 'responds well to visual cues, photographs and symbols and to objects of reference, although he often wants to move to the next activity without taking time to fully understand what is happening and finds waiting a challenge.' She explained that he follows a daily schedule which is sometimes broken down into very small steps.

Cedric can become very anxious quickly if he does not know what he is going to be doing next.

The teacher wanted him to:

- » experience 1:1 time away from the busyness of the classroom;
- » get involved and be encouraged to take some responsibility with the FRT toolkit;
- » experience reflexology, as he generally enjoys positive touch activities; it would be interesting to see how he responds;
- » follow the structure of the session without trying to rush through to finish, as he generally rushes to move on to the next activity;
- » indicate enjoyment of the session when returning to the classroom.

Classroom observation

I had two observation sessions to enjoy activities with Cedric, one in class and one in the playground. It was very helpful to listen to staff instruction and to watch and listen to Cedric seeking attention and how he would ask for adult company and/or for help.

He moved around a lot, he liked to rock on his chair and needed to lift his polo shirt up and down; sometimes he would remove it completely and replace it all within a few seconds. He needed to do this a few times before moving on and continuing to either follow an instruction or to continue with the activity he was already doing.

He liked having individual attention from a member of staff and made it clear he was not happy to share an adult with another pupil.

Before the touch

I used clear communication, reassurance, and calmness of voice. I felt it was helpful that Cedric knew that the calmness of my talking and the clarity I offered was directed at him. I always used his name first and stood where he could see me before I gave him instructions.

Even in the therapy room, when it was only Cedric and me, it was important to begin with his name to focus his attention.

Transition

Visuals can be really helpful for transitions from one activity to another and from the classroom to the therapy room.

Objects of reference

Objects of reference are used to represent an activity, or a person, or an action or event. They are used to share or convey and, importantly, to receive information without using the more conventional form of communication, such as spoken language, sign language, gestures, or pictures.

Reflexology and reflection insights from my records

Cedric found that the FRT toolkit, which I use as an object of reference, helped him to prepare. He began to recognise the bag following the first session. For him, it became a tactile communicative object.

The FRT toolkit is a standardised object of reference that may be meaningful for some and not for others. An additional accessory or object, making it more individual, might be necessary for some young people, so it is important to know the best support for the young person you are working alongside.

For objects of reference to be meaningful, there needs to be an understanding and awareness of the object and what it means. It may also be important not to be too keen to provide too many objects.

On our first visit, I wore a bag and offered Cedric a bag to put on his shoulders, too. Cedric really liked the bag and wanted to get involved. Keen to get the bag on to his shoulders, he did not know on his first visit that it meant we were going to the therapy room. However, as soon as I returned the following week, he was eager to put the bag on and to lead the way to the therapy room. So, for him, this became a super object of reference and encouraged him to get involved in the session before leaving the classroom.

One of the referral targets was about using the toolkit to help foster his understanding.

During the touch

I found my observations helpful in seeing how Cedric responded to visual images and decided to break down the session in the therapy room for the first couple of sessions so Cedric could see what would be happening.

Visual timetable

I created a small picture/symbol board to show the start to the session. Sit down, shoes off, socks off, wipe feet, cream on, music on, lights off, blanket, etc. We used it only for two sessions.

Cedric enjoyed taking the pictures off but I'm not sure we really needed it; I think, in hindsight, my clear, short, verbal instructions and gestures would have been just as meaningful. But it is something to share with the reader, an idea of bringing pictures to help the order of the session. By the way, if you use a visual timetable, it can be designed vertically or horizontally – make it right for the person you are supporting.

The FRT bag became an important part of the session. He often chose to hold on to it during the first few visits to the therapy room. That is, of course, fine. Along with needing the movement of his polo shirt, I think drawing the string of the bag together and pulling it apart helped him settle.

Session 4, 19th March, 2019. I recorded that he dropped the bag over the side of the Lafuma and didn't bother to pick it up. Instead, he placed his hands behind his head. (This was a good moment to look back at in the video following the session.)

After about a minute I stopped my touch just to see what would happen and I signed and asked him if he would like more. Yes, came his sign and he leant forward to pull my hands on to his feet. I took a screenshot from the video and you will see it at the end of the story. The good thing about videos and photos, as I have previously mentioned, is that I can share visual information with staff and parents, and they get to see how both therapist and participant get involved, interact, and work together.

Session 11, 21st May, 2019. One of the wonderful things about documenting in detail and looking back at my records is just how many smiles it has brought me. This one, for example, when all was settled (so I thought): two–three minutes into the session Cedric sat up quickly, then stood up. I waited and watched; he was not upset. I had allowed him to sit and to stand, and he then went on to lift the purple blanket from the hook, no, he changed his mind, he put it on the table and took the red one, and sat down with the chosen blanket.

Yes! I had forgotten to ask or to offer a blanket, so the easiest thing, when he thought about it, was to get up and get his own. I loved that and was very pleased that I did not intervene, just allowed him to sort himself out. It's not always easy at school, or sometimes at home, to encourage and allow independence. Of course, it may also not always be appropriate to allow this, but in the environment of the therapy room, where we have the time and a safe space, it is a good time and place to encourage independence.

Session 13, 11th June, 2019. Another exclamation mark in my records. I wrote, 'settled quickly today and interestingly took my hands to his toes! Cedric gave a deep breath, and he gave lots of smiles, even more than usual. He was noticeably relaxed. I was aware that his usual rapid breathing had slowed very early into the session; I could hear it, but I didn't want to look up. Moving out of sympathetic into parasympathetic.'

After the touch

Cedric loved the 20 minutes of reflexology right from the first session! I often wondered how long he would have sat there for. That could have been an interesting experiment.

As much as he loved the touch it was never a problem finishing the session, with a clear focus and countdown to bring proceedings to an end. I just needed to keep Cedric calm and not to start rushing. I'm not too sure we ever fully achieved this! As soon as we completed the countdown, he would follow me and take in a big breath, then sit up and want socks and shoes on very quickly. He was happy to follow the instruction to replace the towel in the toolkit and always wanted to wear it on his back on the way back to the classroom. But it was always quick, almost 'I've finished this, now what's next?'

So, I encouraged him to look into the toolkit and find an activity (bubbles, squeezy balls, koosh ball, storybook) to continue with while sitting in the Lafuma chair in its upright position. I usually turned the two-minute sandtimer over on the desk next to us. He tolerated it!

Efficacy and effectiveness

Cedric was much more settled when I increased the pressure of the movements. The firm touch on his toes seemed to be a favourite, although I only really became aware of this by watching his facial expression when looking back through the videos. I could see him smiling when his toes where worked, and occasionally looking down towards them.

Teacher feedback

'Cedric is always keen to go with Lorraine. In fact, as soon as he notices she has entered the classroom he wants the bag on his back and can't wait to get on his way.

'Knowing he really enjoyed the session, gave staff a good opportunity to encourage him to wait just a minute, before leaving and to encourage him not try to pull her out of the door. That became a target at the start of the session.

'It was wonderful to have the opportunity to watch some of the video recordings that captured the therapy sessions. Observing Cedric choosing a blanket and getting involved by opening and unpacking the toolkit, taking the towel out and then putting it away at the end again of the session. Lorraine, we really appreciate your introduction of this experience to Cedric. It was good to see him enjoying the time with you and building new connections.'

Feedback from Cedric

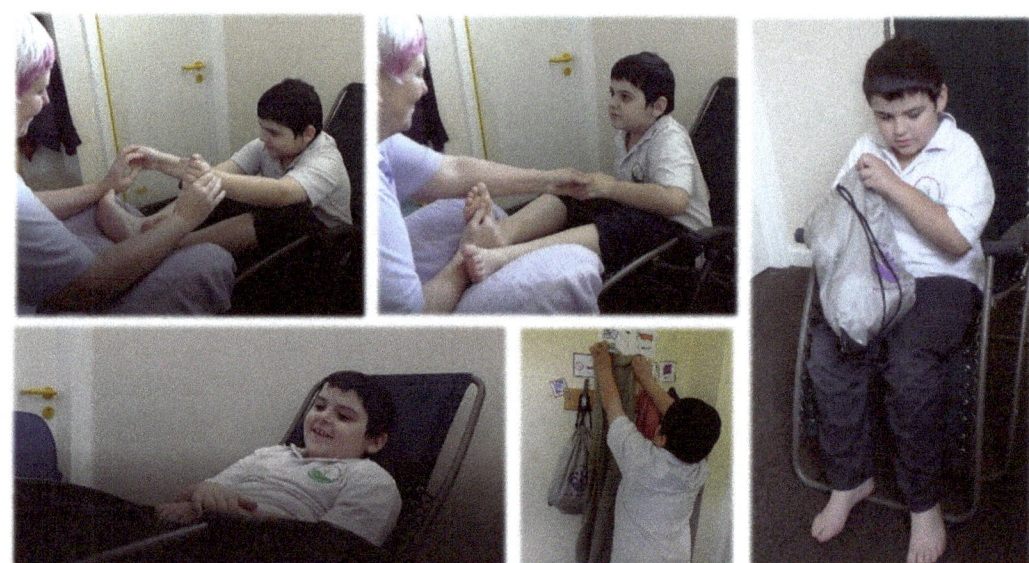

Tips for Reflexologists

» Don't underestimate the power of using the toolkit for communication and enjoyment and the importance of preparation of the young person for the transition of activity.
» Repetition/pressure through full movement and through palpation techniques on the toes was observed to be very calming for Cedric.
» Be an active listener for changes from rapid, shallow breathing to slower, deeper breaths.

Gratitude and Learning

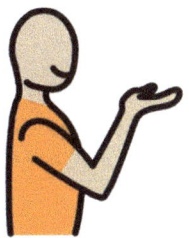

Thank You

Thank you, Cedric, for accepting the invitation to come to the therapy room for reflexology. You have allowed me the opportunity to get to know you just a little bit and not just to work with you. Your participation has helped me to really understand the importance of the support that using objects of reference can bring to enhance the meaningfulness of communication.

Thank you for being the inspiration for the book cover.

Links and Further Information

Global Developmental Delay: www.mencap.org.uk
Objects of reference and communication: www.sense.org.uk
www.sensoryspectacle.co.uk

Chapter 14: Meet Kayleigh

'I love looking in the toolkit at the end of the session, especially when I find the bubbles.'

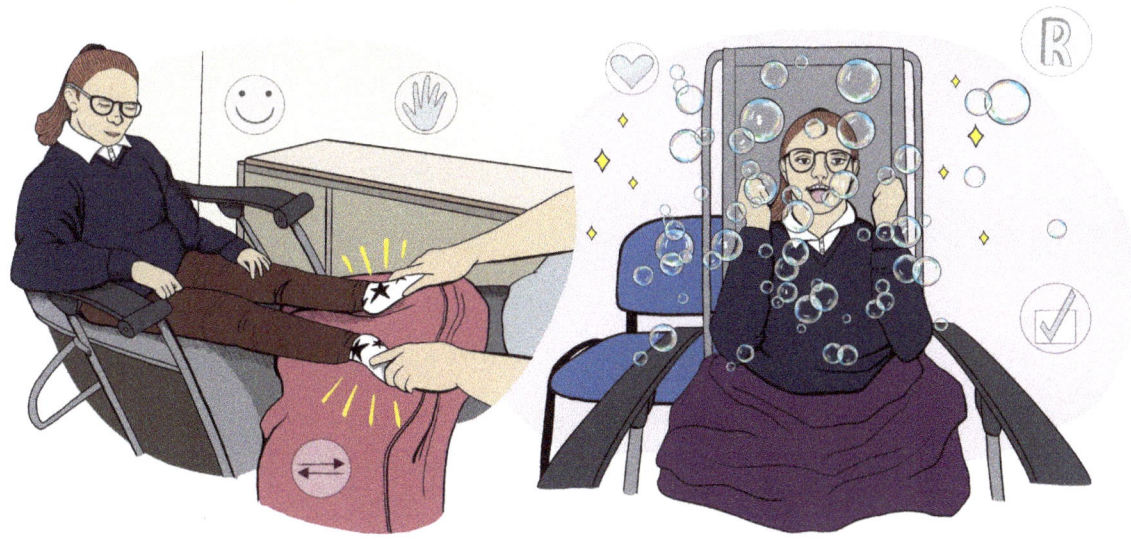

OUR WORK BEGAN together in December 2021 when Kayleigh was 13 years of age.

Kayleigh thoroughly enjoys engaging with adults and her friends in the classroom. She is generally very smiley and very interested to see everything that is going on around her.

Kayleigh has a diagnosis of 1p36 deletion syndrome, including delayed speech and language skills. This is a congenital genetic disorder characterised by moderate to severe intellectual disability and delayed growth.

The Process

Teacher referral

This followed the annual review and professional discussion in which mum expressed concern about Kayleigh refusing touch, not just from medical professionals but also when needing her fingernails and toenails cut, and said health and hygiene was becoming an issue. The teacher discussed the possibility of inviting Kayleigh for some fun in the therapy room with the intention of her accepting positive touch and beginning to tolerate it.

The teacher asked if the therapy session could help to reduce her anxiety about touch and be supportive with the issue raised in the annual review.

Hypersensitivity

Kayleigh is hypersensitive, particularly with regard to touch, where she seems to dislike physical contact. Perhaps she finds it uncomfortable. Hypersensitivity could also mean being highly sensitive to all things physical through sound, sight, and smell, as well as touch.

The teacher wanted her to:

- settle into the therapy sessions with the intention of reducing feelings of anxiousness when receiving touch;
- offering her consent to have feet and hands touched so she begins to feel in control of the activity;
- develop a trust for touch that may be transferable to other situations (for example the doctor or dentist);
- take a little responsibility for using the toolkit and to engage and get involved in the session;
- to have the opportunity and time to use her signing skills to enjoy communication in the therapy room;
- support well-being issues highlighted by her parent;
- develop awareness of her own hygiene and care for hands and feet.

On receiving the referral, I discussed with the class teacher what I felt I could bring to the therapy session to support Kayleigh and how I felt I could work towards addressing the parent's concerns raised in the review.

The session to support Kayleigh would need to be carefully structured 'beyond the touch' to create a fun environment while working towards addressing the objectives to encourage her to tolerate the touch.

Classroom observation

Although I was already familiar with Kayleigh and she with me, it was good to spend a session in the classroom with Kayleigh signing and chattering. It helped me to focus on a small number of signs to use in the therapy room. Generally, Kayleigh was very happy, but I did see a more stubborn or determined side. So, I felt if Kayleigh was unhappy about the session and did not like coming to the therapy room, she was going to let me know and she would make it very clear to the classroom!

Reflexology and reflection insights from my records

I introduced myself with my photograph and the FRT bag, which was over my shoulder. The photograph could remain with Kayleigh for her timetable. I offered the bag to Kayleigh. It was a great success from the first session. She signalled that she wanted it on her back, and I feel it helped her with her preparation. It was a super communicative support for her, helping her to feel that she was involved and taking some responsibility.

She knew where she was going and what she would be doing. She is already familiar with the use of a backpack as she brings one to school and takes out her home schoolbook and snacks on arrival.

Fun

This was always going to be an interesting challenge as the main intention was to encourage Kayleigh to accept, tolerate, and possibly even enjoy, touch on her feet. If Kayleigh is hypersensitive to the touch, particularly on her feet, it could be very overwhelming and uncomfortable and, as mentioned by her mum, it has become a very difficult issue, particularly at home.

I needed to invite Kayleigh to a fun yet calm environment and create the right space. There was work to be done but I needed Kayleigh to enjoy the session and perhaps choose some activities that she may like at the end of the session.

In the first session Kayleigh followed my request to remove shoes and socks and pointed to the underneath of the big toe on her left foot. I thought I knew what she was showing me, but I needed the school nurse to confirm and to inform home. (*Reflexologists, remember your responsibilities and boundaries; you are not there to diagnose but to inform and seek medical support, even if you feel you know.*) The nurse confirmed a cluster of verrucae.

Session 2, 7th December, 2021. Kayleigh decided she would not take her socks off and told me in no uncertain terms!

Perhaps there was some discomfort, and this could be one reason that she was very hesitant. But if she was happy to remove her shoes, I decided I would start with some central solar plexus techniques and lower leg touch, reassuringly away from the toes.

During the first few weeks, Kayleigh was offered a choice of chair, firm and upright or the large, softer chair that I could alter in angle and position. Kayleigh chose to sit in the Lafuma but preferred it to remain in an upright position. She would remove her shoes on request.

Socks remained on for several weeks and the chair remained upright. I would always start with the same instruction, shoes off, socks off, and Kayleigh would choose, and we would have a little fun each week reclining the chair a tiny bit. She giggled a lot; we were both enjoying the session and each week we managed a little bit more touch.

Session 7, 22nd February, 2022. I used the term 'flying' as we reclined the chair. She loved it, instantly flapping her arms as the chair slowly reclined and we had to repeat it several times. This became the general beginning of the session and from this session on, she has seemed to really enjoy having the chair reclined and the action of 'flying' back.

Session 18, 5th July, 2022. The important note here is the length of timing of the session. The touch time had increased to 12 minutes. (Touch time in session one was approximately two minutes.)

It wasn't just about tolerance; she appeared to be enjoying the touch along the inside of each foot with the repetition of the rhythmic circling motion supporting the spine area and central nervous system (CNS). During this movement I noticed she would often stop chatting, stop giggling, and be still, and sometimes look down towards her feet and occasionally sit up and look more closely.

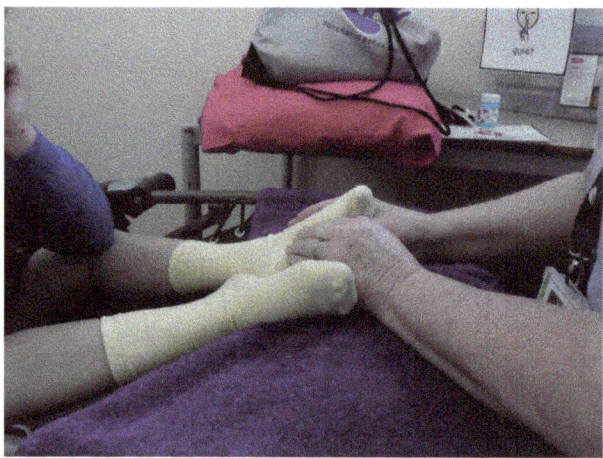

To end the session, I wanted something fun in the toolkit. Kayleigh and I sat together to choose two activities to put in the toolkit. One was a book and the other was the bubbles. Sometimes, in the early sessions, she liked to hold the book and show me a few pictures, but the bubbles were always a choice for the end of the session. Lots of popping fun and giggles and using some signing, enjoying communication together.

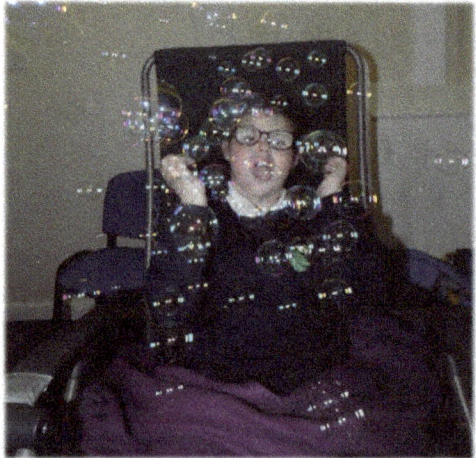
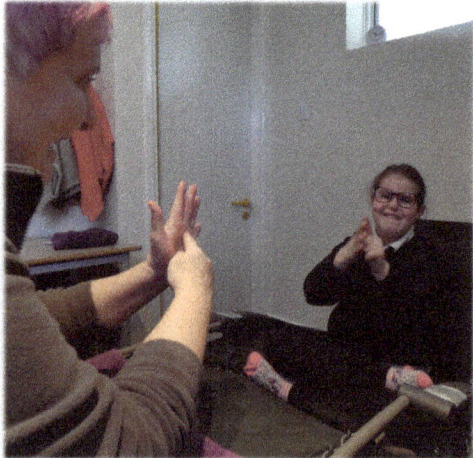

Efficacy and effectiveness

The touch time had increased from two minutes to 12 minutes. This had to be an enjoyable experience for Kayleigh to help to build tolerance of touch and support mum with personal care. Of course, this is not reflexology as we reflexologists would know it, but it is using some very specific rhythmically delivered reflexology techniques for calmness and to allow Kayleigh to become more comfortable with the touch.

This highlights the importance and value of using the skills of a reflexologist supported with FRT as part of the multidisciplinary team during the school day.

Teacher feedback

'Kayleigh always returns with a smile, so we know she is enjoying the fun in the therapy room and the one-to-one adult attention, usually entering the classroom just before snack time with the FRT bag on her back, she is quick to give it back to Lorraine to let her know she has finished with a wave goodbye.'

The teacher commented that the classroom staff all love to see the independence on returning to the classroom.

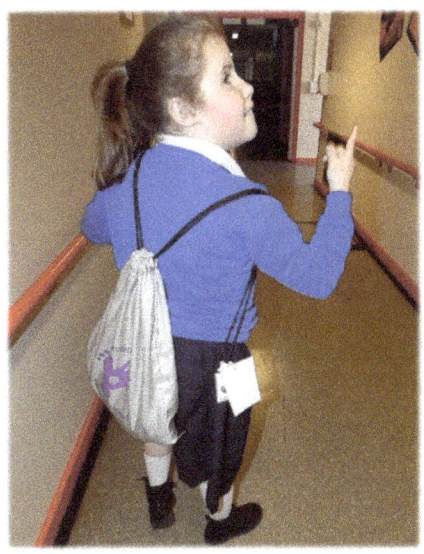
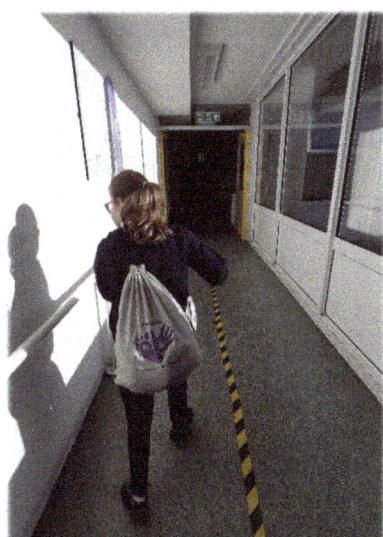

'It is also really nice to see Kayleigh signing the L for Lorraine and pointing to her feet on the morning she sees it on her timetable.'

Parent feedback

'I am really pleased that this opportunity was discussed during the annual review and the school have been able to find time for Kayleigh to have this experience during the school day.

'I can read through feedback and see from Lorraine usually in the form of nice photos that Kayleigh is enjoying the sessions and is allowing some touch to her feet. I think it will take a long time for her to comfortably allow personal care of her feet if ever.

'It has made a difference working with Lorraine. Kayleigh is enjoying time with her sister painting her nails, this never used to happen.'

Tips for Reflexologists

- Remember, the 'tiniest' steps can take a long time but are so very important and are major achievements.
- Your therapy can be as beneficial with socks on as it is with socks off! Always consider the value and what you are trying to work towards.
- Involve the nurse with health and hygiene information and raise awareness of verrucae, which could be done as a whole school informative leaflet.

Feedback from Kayleigh

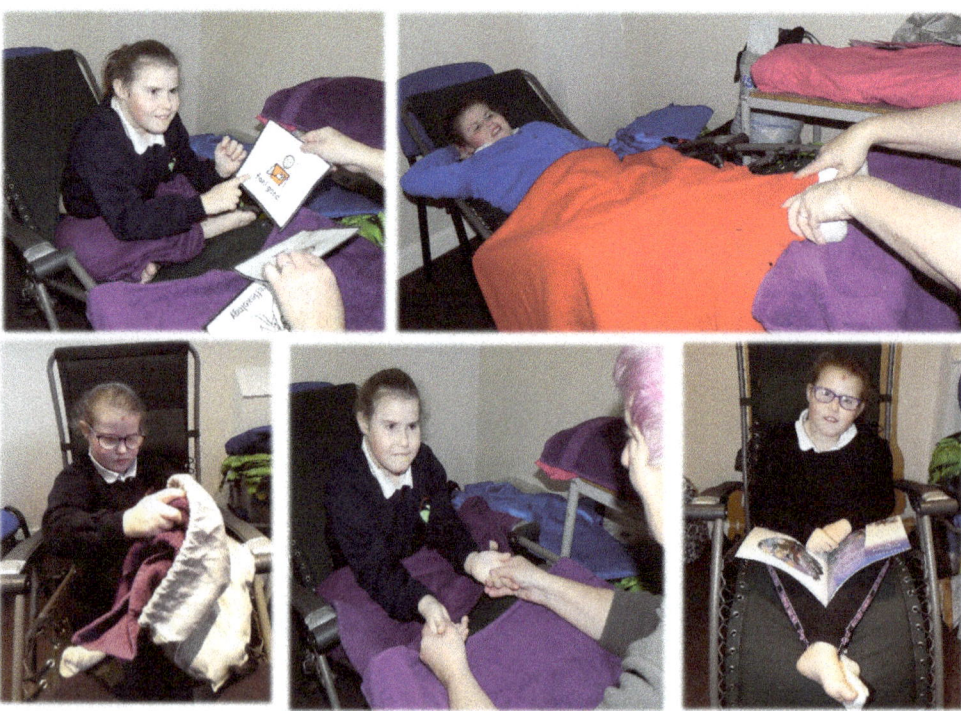

Gratitude and Learning

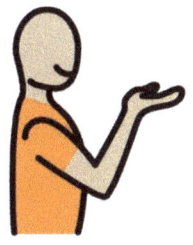

Thank You

Thank you, Kayleigh, for accepting the invitation to come to the therapy room for reflexology. You have allowed me the opportunity to get to know you a little bit, and you have helped me with my Makaton signing. We have had lots of enjoyable moments, even if I'm not always sure what we have been laughing about, but it has been fun.

Links and Further Information

1p36 deletion syndrome is a disorder:	www.rarechromo.org
Makaton, language programme:	www.makaton.org
Verrucas and warts:	www.nhs.uk/conditions/warts-and-verrucas/

Chapter 15: Meet Dan

'I love all the movements, but I particularly like the circles on my toes.'

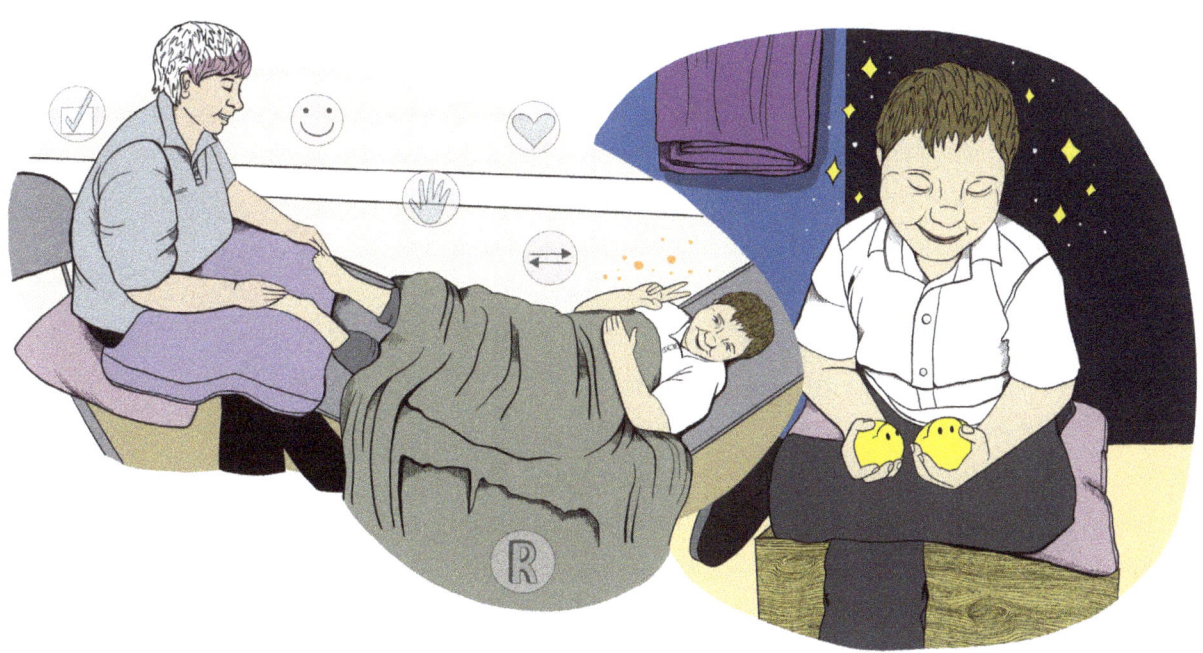

OUR WORK TOGETHER began in 2012 when Dan was eight years of age.

Dan has a warm, smiley, and vibrant presence. He enjoys welcoming everyone and always seems pleased to see you. He seems to love an opportunity to engage with most people with his outgoing nature and really enjoys being involved.

Dan has Down's syndrome and severe learning difficulties; he needs support and individual approaches to help him to understand and learn new skills, and to help him with his communication and support him to express his feelings and emotions.

The Process

Teacher referral

Dan's teacher wrote that on occasions he found things very frustrating and used behaviours that were not appropriate to try to get attention in the classroom, and, although he seems very sociable, it can be challenging to understand each other at times.

At the time I began working with Dan he was taking strong medication for the discomfort he was suffering through juvenile arthritis and would rarely sleep more than three–four hours a night. The medication side-effects and his sleep difficulties were significantly affecting his attendance at school and, when he was able to attend, the teacher had considered that his lack of sleep, fatigue, and discomfort may be affecting his focus and how he was managing his emotions throughout the school day.

The teacher asked, if Dan was to receive reflexology, could it help to relax, to ease discomfort and possibly help with his sleep issues.

The teacher wanted him to:

- » experience a new sensory therapy, being able to make the choice if he wanted to attend or not;
- » have an opportunity to build a new relationship;
- » have the opportunity to accept the touch and show calmness and relaxation from receiving it;
- » indicate his enjoyment (or not) and likes or dislikes of the session when returning to the classroom;
- » explore if the therapy could help with him with regulation of sleep;
- » explore if the therapy could help to reduce any discomfort due to the juvenile arthritis.

Classroom observation

It was helpful to take my observation into the classroom. I could see that generally Dan was very sociable, and keen to join in with everything. It was evident that he thrived on adult attention. But also, there were moments of 'stubbornness', and when he decided not to do something, he was not going to do it! It was interesting and very helpful for me to watch the strategies that were used to encourage him.

I felt confident that he would like the time away from class, but it would be interesting to discover if he was going to enjoy the touch.

Reflexology and reflection insights from my records

Before I sent information about reflexology and consent letters home, I invited Dan to the therapy room to have a look around, with the aim for him to familiarise himself with the room and the equipment. He really liked the toolkit, emptying out its contents and repacking them. He sat in the large chair, and rather liked it when it reclined, and he listened to some music.

It was clear, early on, that Dan loved using the FRT toolkit. He carried it down to the therapy room and was keen to get involved and prepare the space and himself. He removed the towel, popped it on to the pillow and spent time pushing the creases out and flattening it. He looked for the balm and the spatula, which he took great pleasure in handing to me.

There was some absenteeism in the early weeks, which was bound to affect becoming familiar, and it might have been this that influenced how settled Dan was. But as the graph below shows, each session increased in the length of the touch time from the initial eight minutes on 7th November, 2012, to 15 minutes by 27th February, 2013.

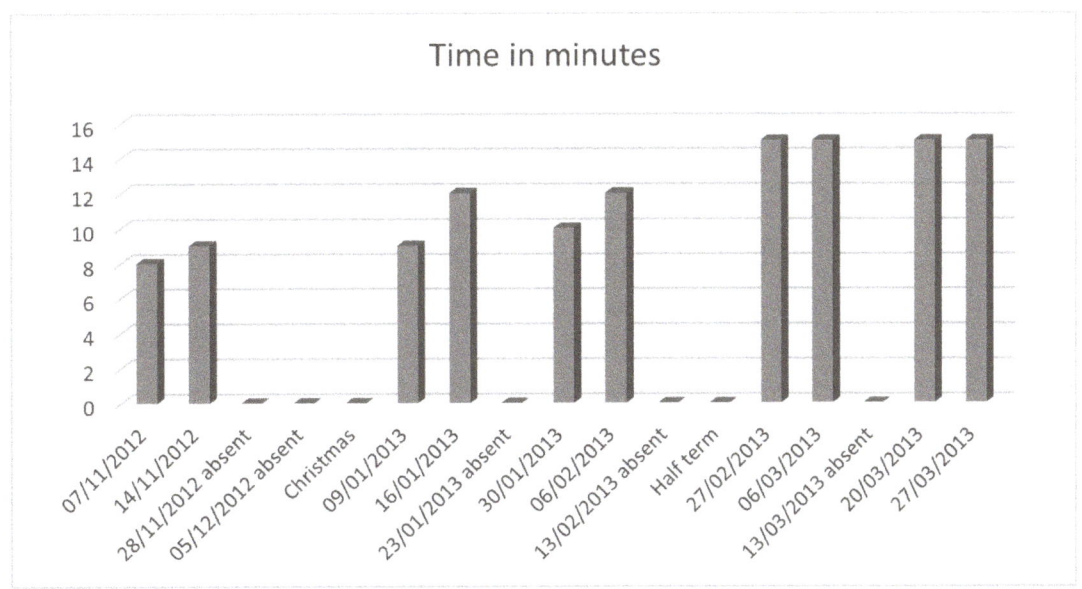

A graph showing the increase of touch time

For Dan, 30 minutes out of class and 15 minutes touch time worked well. The sessions were achieving their objective.

Efficacy and effectiveness

As the weekly sessions continued, Dan was still talkative and chatty, but he would occasionally close his eyes and there were moments of smiles and silence. I know he was generally tired during the school day; it wasn't my intention to encourage him to sleep but for his body to be calm and to ease the busyness of his mind.

My notes consistently mention a warmth felt in his toes and around his ankles and at times the whole of his feet and ankles felt quite warm, perhaps a symptom of general inflammation throughout his body and sometimes they looked and felt quite puffy.

6th February, 2013. I recorded the heat of his feet, and he mentioned a few times 'sore'. He did not remove them. I asked 'Is it okay to touch? Do you want more reflexology?' He said yes.

He was okay with me holding his toes, both feet at the same time, and using a small pulsing technique to provide a rhythmical movement on his toes while gently swaying his feet from side to side. I was watching for any changes in skin colour, feeling any changes in temperature, and actively listening to any quietening of his voice and length of stillness time.

The touch was proving very enjoyable and was very well received, and Dan absolutely loved the sessions. He got comfortable preparing himself, settled, and chatted lots about anything! The challenge arrived at the end of the session, we would count down, both take a good big breath, and I would return the chair to its upright position. Then came the stubbornness.

Using the toolkit

And so ... the stubbornness. Well, to me, it was a 'terrific' stubbornness, more like a little cheekiness. Socks on, NO, shoes on, NO! It was almost as if he wanted to tell me, 'I'm having such a lovely time I don't want it to stop.' However, it was the end of the session, so he had to learn to respect that, too.

My response was to find a strategy beyond the touch that did not involve firm instruction. I did not want to change the calm atmosphere that had been created within the therapy room, so it needed to be something that might tempt Dan out of the chair to play 'once' he has his socks and shoes on ... Aaahhh! This is when the squeezy balls arrived! And FUN!

Interestingly, these have a second supportive role, too, as mentioned with Harley – counting up, squeezing, and supporting the solar plexus area to aid calm and focus.

6th March, 2013. My records read, 'Dan's best session yet.' I note the touch time had increased to 15 minutes for the second week in a row. He independently put his socks and shoes on, walked quietly back to the classroom, stopped at the water fountain in the upper school corridor for a quick slurp and entered his classroom, telling everyone with a big smile and in a big voice, 'I'm back.'

12th June, 2013. I recorded that Dan came into school late, as he had had a poor night's sleep. The teacher felt the start to the day had unsettled him. I went to meet him in the playground to invite him for reflexology and I noted that I got a grumpy welcome.

I gave him a little time to think about coming along and let him to know that he had a choice. I waited, and chatted to some children. He gave it some thought, came over to take the toolkit from my shoulder, and we continued as usual. Dan looked in the toolkit at the end of the session for the squeezy balls and we did some extra squeezing and breathing. This has really improved and it's great that they became part of his FRT toolkit to end the session.

Teacher feedback

'We love it when Dan comes back into the lesson after a session with Lorraine, it truly doesn't matter what we are doing, he comes in with a big smile and lets everyone know he is in a good mood. I cannot recall a time he has not enjoyed it.'

The teacher said that he will settle into work on return, but he does like to talk a little about what he did in the session, and that he will often mention sitting in the big chair and lying down.

Feedback from Dan

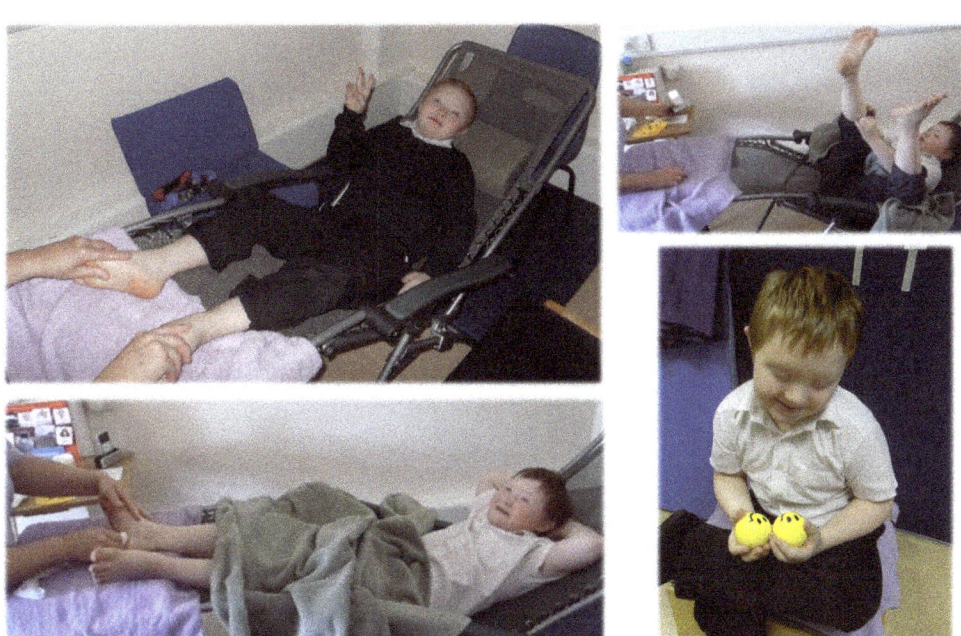

Tips for Reflexologists

» Do not underestimate the value of getting the young person involved in the session. The therapy session begins when you collect from the classroom.
» Be flexible and adapt your techniques. Every technique is delivered with the same intent, to calm, to settle, to balance, to relax. Try working with bi-manual support of the toes, to balance and calm the mind.
» Consider what might work as a motivator in your toolkit, if your young client doesn't want to finish or get out of the chair. You might need clear communication, a structure after completing your touch and a fun selection.

At the time of the writing of this book, I do not work with individual sessions with Dan, but, throughout the past few years, he has enjoyed whole class group self-care sessions. He follows the movements through the FRT Rainbow Relaxation Routine on his own hands, he changes from one movement to another and is great at taking long slow breaths.

Lorraine Senior

As of March 2023, it is over ten years since we first started our work together. We often meet in the corridor during our days, and he will greet me with a surprised expression, Oh it's you! He always brings me a smile and he will check when I will next be visiting the classroom.

The Dan I meet now is polite, still very smiley, and, I love to use the word, jolly. He is currently enjoying work experience during time in the sixth form, and he is happy for me to share his up-to-date self-care photograph.

My hope for Dan is that he continues to enjoy and use the self-care rainbow routine, especially now he has a copy of the supportive 15-minute video to play in his own time to support his own well-being as he moves forward, and I wish Dan lots of luck.

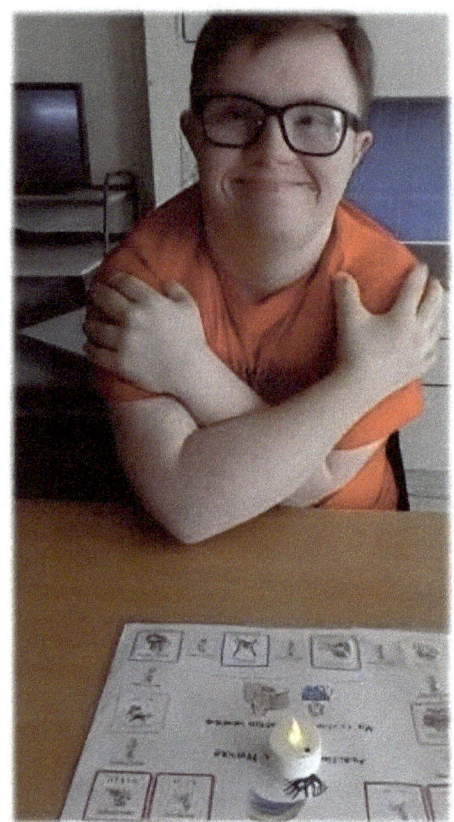

Gratitude and Learning

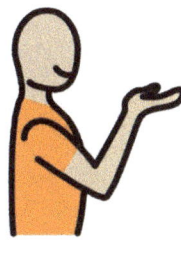

Thank You

Thank you, Dan, for accepting the invitation to join me in the therapy room for reflexology. Thank you for being such fun and allowing me to get to know you a little bit. While I was supporting you, I studied to learn more about some of the challenges you may be working with, such as with juvenile arthritis. It really helped me to consider how I delivered some of the reflexology techniques.

Your 'stubbornness' in not wanting the reflexology session to finish always brought me a smile although I couldn't show you that! I needed to think about motivators to encourage you to get out of the chair to replace your socks and shoes. I discovered your love for the squeezy balls, which I could hide in the FRT toolkit, and that they were very effective for this transition purpose.

Links and Further Information

Down's Syndrome Association: www.downs-syndrome.org.uk
Juvenile Arthritis: www.arthritis.org/diseases/juvenile-arthritis

Chapter 16: Meet Suzzie

'I smile when Lorraine does a rocking movement on my ankles. The whole chair bounces.'

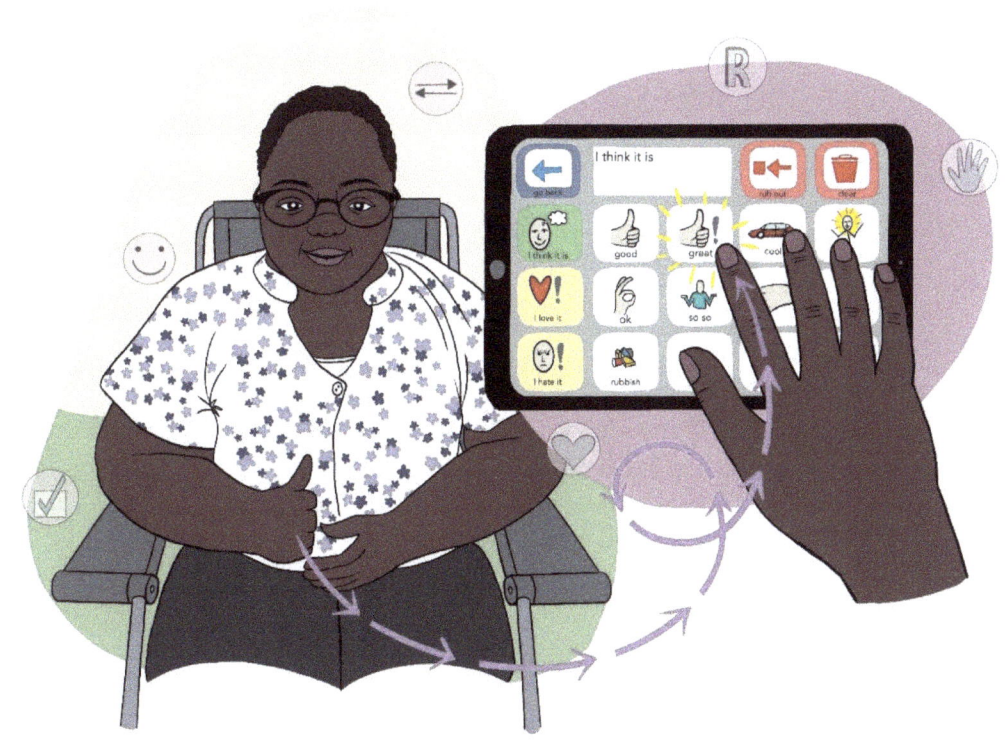

OUR WORK TOGETHER began in November 2021 when Suzzie was 16 years of age.

Suzzie possesses a very quiet, shy outward appearance at school and when her smile arrives it is delightful and a special moment, almost as if she has been trying to hold it back and it has broken out! Just allowing herself to 'be in the moment' she shares a little glimpse of the real Suzzie.

Suzzie has Trisomy 21 Down's syndrome, hypothyroidism, learning difficulties, significant speech difficulty, severe communication difficulties (non-speaking) diagnosed with suspected insulin resistance, with a severe vision impairment.

Suzzie is making progress with skills to use her iPad to support her communication and to give her a voice. Suzzie will very occasionally use some words in a very quiet voice, although this has become less frequent in recent years.

The Process

Teacher referral

The teacher thought Suzzie would enjoy the quiet environment of the therapy room and the sensory experience of foot reflexology, and wondered if receiving one-to-one personal attention may give her the opportunity for time to relax and allow her to express how she is feeling and communicate if she feels able to and if she chooses to.

The teacher would like her to:

- » experience time away from the busyness of the classroom;
- » enjoy the sensory experience;
- » be given time and opportunity to express how she is feeling;
- » be encouraged to make choices and express preferences;
- » understand she has the choice to go for reflexology or not;
- » know she can stop the touch when in the therapy room at any time and have an appropriate method of communication available.

Classroom observation

I enjoyed one observation with Suzzie before she began the sessions. She occasionally lifted her head to look around. She sat very still and quiet, slowly followed the instructions given by the teacher and staff. She was given lots of encouragement and time to get on with her work. During my observation there was no direct social interaction between Suzzie and staff or other pupils.

I had taken some photographs of the therapy room and took the FRT toolkit to show Suzzie. We shared some time together, we looked at what was inside the bag, and I talked about what would happen in the therapy room.

Suzzie came for a visit to look in the therapy room, and I showed her the reclining chair. I sat in it, and she watched me lie back. I asked her if she would like to have a go. I stood at her side and placed my hand on her right shoulder as the chair began to recline. I could tell she was very apprehensive; her eye movements were rapid, and she placed her hands on the arms of the Lafuma. But I felt that the placement of my hand on her shoulder and how I used my voice, calmly and quietly, was reassuring and I continued with the recline.

The intention at this point was to show and share information to help Suzzie to understand what was being offered.

It was very helpful for me to work alongside the speech and language therapist (SLT) for ideas to bring into the FRT framework to support my reflexology session. Using the iPad as a meaningful method of communication was crucial for Suzzie.

Getting involved

I take the FRT bag to the classroom and ask Suzzie if she would like to come along for reflexology. She replies after a minute or two by checking the top of her water bottle and placing it in the FRT bag along with her iPad.

She usually turns, ready for the bag to be popped over her shoulders, and off we go to the therapy room.

I am usually positive with my words: for example, 'Good to see you', and will often indicate my joy at the colours she is wearing.

It is always a quiet walk; Suzzie walks very slowly and sometimes links her arm through mine.

To this date, Suzzie has not been able to share any spoken word with me on the way, in the therapy room, or on the way back, but we have shared a few beautiful smiles.

Reflexology and reflection insights from my records

I always offer a choice of blanket; we have four different colours in the therapy room and Suzzie likes to alternate between red and purple. At the time of writing this, Suzzie was still coming along for weekly sessions and purple seemed to be her favourite.

Session 8, 12th January, 2022. I have noticed that, as the weeks have progressed, so has Suzzie's subtle confidence on arrival.

- » She was starting to push the door open and walk into the therapy room on arrival rather than waiting for me to give her permission or for me do it for her.
- » She makes a choice of music by looking at the CD covers. I have three and it brings a tiny movement of her lips, may be a little smile, when I say 'Oooh, you had the blue tranquillity last week and this week you have chosen the green chillout.'
- » While I am putting the music on, she will now begin to prepare herself to take off her shoes and socks rather than waiting for the instruction.

I continue to use the CD player rather than the technology of my phone or bluetooth speaker because I think you lose the visual understanding, seeing the coloured cases, giving an option to choose. I suppose over time it will change as CDs disappear. Maybe I will have to print out pictures to represent different choices.

Session 15, 27th April, 2022. We had been using the iPad at the end of the sessions and Suzzie was telling me that it was good. She would answer the question 'Would you like to come back next week?'

Allowing time

Allowing time to process the question being asked and sufficient time to give an answer is important.

Efficacy and effectiveness

On the way back to the classroom following the session, Suzzie has a better walking position and lifts her feet a little higher. There is not quite as much of a shuffle to her movement.

You might or might not know that hypothyroidism can cause extreme anxiety. It can affect the body in so many ways. The NHS support site states it can include nervousness, anxiety, it can affect a person's mood and can cause much tiredness. Think about those symptoms and the effect it may have on Suzzie during the school day, her desire to join in, and her frame of mind for learning.

Can I, as the reflexologist, offer her an enjoyable, supportive session that may help her to cope better throughout the day by showing kindness and care with a different approach?

We have established together, through questions, smiles, movements, and use of the iPad, that Suzzie likes to have both feet worked on at the same time, working both feet and legs simultaneously.

Teacher feedback

'Sometimes it is difficult to gauge how Suzzie is feeling but we can see when she walks back into the classroom her head is held quite high and I know she has given Lorraine feedback about liking the session.'

Before the next session, at some point in the week, a member of staff will refer to reflexology and ask Suzzie, using her iPad if she does enjoy going for the session and if she would like to go the following week.

Feedback from Suzzie

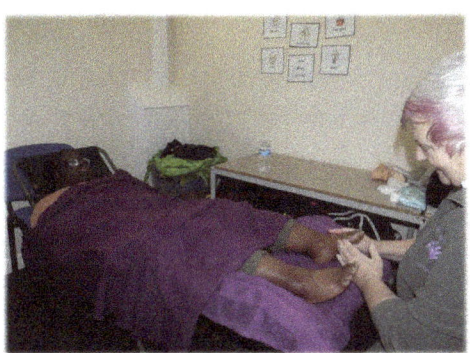
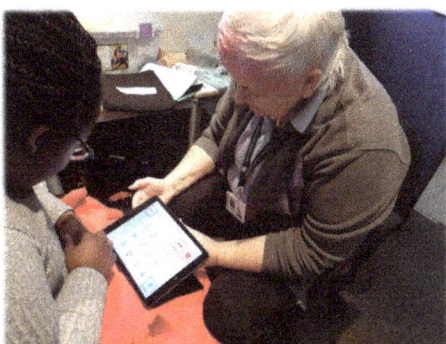
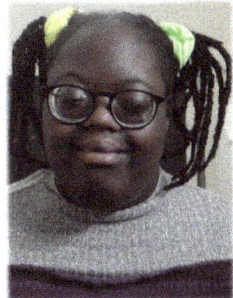
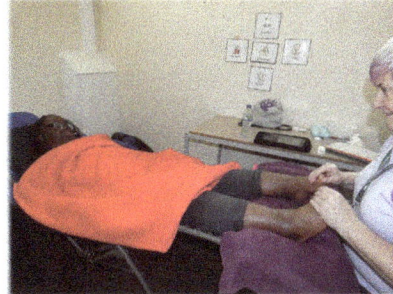
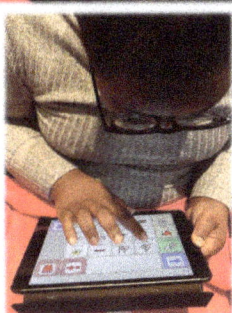

> ### Tips for Reflexologists
>
> » It is important to gather as much information as possible from the team and parents. Remember you are not 'treating' one condition, but looking at the overall intention to help the participant to be in a better frame of mind.
> » Diaphragm rocking technique (Lynne Booth method) works well alongside the diaphragm stretch technique, repeating the sweeping linking movement, encouraging a few big breaths through the stretches.
> » Work alongside class teacher and speech and language therapist to support communication and use a communication aid in a meaningful way.

Suzzie has many medical conditions, so it's important to gather as much information as possible. If the reflexologist has questions or concerns, talk to the school nurse, or do some extra research.

Undoubtedly, these sessions offered valuable support through the nurturing touch of reflexology, working alongside the team that is offering and encouraging Suzzie with other interventions and opportunities.

Kindness, caring, relaxation, one-to-one attention and, importantly, the provision of time allowed Suzzie the space to make choices, to make her own decisions, and share her feedback.

Gratitude and Learning

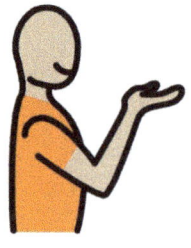

Thank You

Thank you, Suzzie, for accepting the invitation to come to the therapy room for reflexology. You have allowed me the opportunity to get to know you just a little bit and not just to work with you. You have helped me to watch and listen for subtle hand and facial gestures valuable for respectful communication and development of meaningful connections. I feel these sessions were very supportive and empowering for you.

Links and Further Information

Professional body for Speech and Language Therapy: www.rcslt.org
Speech and Language Therapy AAC: www.slt.co.uk

Chapter 17: Meet Fred

'I like the sweeping movements on my legs, it makes me laugh, but my real favourite is when Lorraine gently squeezes my foot and hand at the same time.'

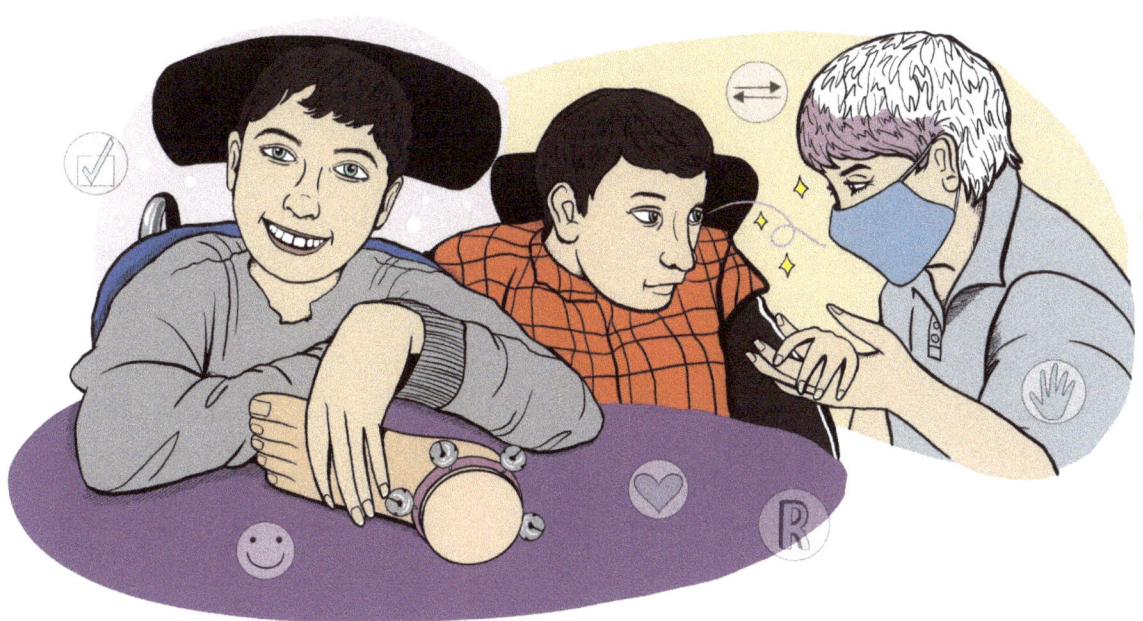

OUR WORK TOGETHER began in September 2021 when Fred was 16 years of age, and, as you probably remember, it was at a particularly challenging time in our lives when the world became familiar with partially covering the face. It brought different stresses into already challenging individual lives. Fred continued to lean forward towards the voice. I wonder how its sound through the mask changed for him and what he thought about not feeling any warm breath, or whether he might prefer the covering.

Although Fred does not use words, he has plenty to say. He uses many different sounds and body language: lifting his head, stretching out his arm and shaking some noisy equipment or knocking it on his tray to get adult attention all share how he is feeling. He has a beautiful smile and uses it to communicate agreement and a way to give consent or a way to indicate that he is not in agreement and does not give consent.

Fred has cerebral palsy, is severely visually impaired, with profound and multiple learning difficulties (PMLD), and has a diagnosis of epilepsy. Fred has a shunt which helps to drain excess fluid from his brain. He is wheelchair dependent. The term PMLD is not a diagnosis, but is a term used to describe a person who has one or more disabilities. A person that is described as having PMLD may have difficulties with communicating, learning or sensory disabilities, complex health needs, and challenges with their independence.

The Process

Listen to the silence, it can say so much

Fred communicates with sounds, objects, with his movements, noises, and gestures and he does have a lot to say. Even his stillness has a valuable meaning.

I wonder how often you have given thought to how some communication challenges and health difficulties also bring fear, anger, and sadness. Fred will often express fret and frustration through his sounds and through the tension throughout his body. The energy that he uses just to communicate is exhausting – it's no wonder he gets frustrated.

Have you ever taken time to consider just how much daily energy is needed to communicate where great effort and exertion is required to listen, to process and understand, and then to work out how to respond and then communicate the response? It has such a huge impact on the quality of time and energy used during the school day.

At what point does he say, 'Enough is enough, I'm fed up, it's so hard, I can't be bothered, you don't understand what I am saying, so I'll shout loudly, or I'll grumble, or I'll cry, or do you know what – I'll just remain quiet and then everything can just continue on around me and I'm not bothering anyone and I can gather a little energy.'

Teacher referral

The teacher wanted Fred to be given the opportunity for reflexology to enjoy the positive touch in a quiet environment.

The teacher wanted him to:

» experience time away from the busyness of the classroom to have a quiet 1:1 adult positive touch session;
» be provided with appropriate communicative methods to have the opportunity to make decisions;
» have a session that might encourage him to express his feelings;

- » be helped to understand about his right to give consent to touch;
- » be helped to understand that he is in control of the session and can stop at any time.
- » have well-being issues highlighted by parents supported;
- » be given the opportunity to indicate enjoyment (or not) of the session when returning to the classroom.

Classroom observation

I am fortunate to have been supporting the classroom team with the positive touch of the Rainbow Relaxation Activity during the past few years, so I do feel I have got to know Fred a little.

It is so important that he is given the opportunity to have his say and allow him a voice, and he is offered a small selection of meaningful objects of reference. He likes tactility and noise, the sound of banging something on his tray and possibly the vibration sensation he receives, and changes in the voice addressing him, as you will read later.

Although Fred was already familiar with me, it was still important that I helped him to understand that I was inviting him for something new. He is used to the FRT Rainbow Relaxation Programme in the classroom, so I know he loves the touch, but he needed to know that the session I was going to be inviting him to would be similar but different, and it was going to take place in a different part of the school.

We went to the therapy room. I played music that I planned to use each week, we took a little time to settle, to listen, look at and feel the toolkit, which I hoped would help Fred to begin to familiarise himself with the new upcoming activity.

Gauging music preference is difficult. How do I know he likes it? I know that he likes the reflexology and coming along for the sessions. The addition of music is another form of communication to introduce the session. I tested turning the music on and off during the therapy but I did not recognise any noticeable impact, any likes or dislikes. The music might bring an initial awareness but is perhaps not necessary in the therapy room. The touch and my voice seemed much more influential and meaningful for Fred.

Remember the R E C I P E: developing meaningful connections, communication enhancing awareness, understanding and preparation and be respectful of what works and what is appropriate and/or necessary.

Fred's toolkit and objects of reference are the towel, my greeting with balm on the hand, some initial music, perhaps the bells around the foot model, but, importantly, my voice.

Aroma

Whether you use a balm or a cream during reflexology is a personal choice – not everyone likes it. However, if you do use a balm or cream, I recommend that you use an unscented brand. There are some key points to bear in mind. If you choose to use an aroma in the school setting or any setting when you are supporting someone who may find it very difficult to express likes and dislikes and preferences, there are a few important points here for you to consider.

- » Do you understand how the body may react to specific smells and their triggers?
- » Personal preferences will definitely vary.
- » If someone can express a preference and you use their choice, what happens when that aroma is still in the room and the next person comes in who really does not like it?
- » Beware of any active ingredients in the balm and potential effects to the skin.
- » Some reflexologists work with talcum powder. This is an absolutely *must not* in the school setup. Respiratory risk assessment for the use of any powder is mandatory and best avoided.

If at all daunted, undecided or unsure, don't worry, just don't use it! You can deliver your amazing touch on top of socks or tights or directly on to the skin without any type of cream, balm, or oil.

However, you may choose to use an aroma to indicate your session as a way of communicating. You could consider putting a natural aroma into a vial, test tube, or small jar so that you can offer the aroma and replace the lid to contain the smell away from others. Talk to the teacher and find out what they use for any olfactory work.

Reflexology and reflection insights from my records

I always start, with a clear introduction in the classroom. 'Hello Fred, it's Lorraine here. I have brought the reflexology bag, let's open the bag together and find out what is inside.'

He might squeeze the bag, he might hold the foot model that has some bells around it – he rather likes the sound it makes by banging it on his tray. However, he usually responds most to my voice. I bend down close to one side and talk clearly, not too loudly. I say it is time for reflexology and ask him if he is ready for the sweep, using my voice to signal sweeping uuuuup and sweeping doooown (hope you get the gist here). Sometimes I need to wait a while for him to respond, which is usually a giggle and/or a smile and I feel reassured he has recognised me, and he is preparing.

Waiting is important so that he knows he is in control of this session; we do not leave the classroom until Fred has let me know he is ready. Using some multi-sensory methods can really help with awareness for transitions.

As soon as we leave the classroom, Fred's demeanour changes, he does not seem unhappy in the classroom, but he absolutely loves coming out and knowing he has 1:1 attention. His sounds change and get louder, and he will often lift his head up.

Fred is generally happy and alert; however, there are moments when he might feel tired or be experiencing discomfort somewhere and he can be very quiet, or very loud, his sounds do differ. Every sound is a type of communication, something he wants to share. I often consult staff who have spent significant time with him during the day or throughout the week to help me understand more.

It's also important to mention here the value of picking up information from staff when you go into the classroom. It could be valuable for your session approach.

Sometimes Fred's socks are on, sometimes they are off, sometimes I work just the feet, sometimes I work just the hands, sometimes I work the hands and feet one after the other and sometimes I work the hands and feet synergistically. (Synergistic reflexology is a term introduced by Lynne Booth, creator of Vertical Reflex Therapy, tutor, and reflexologist.) It involves working the same reflex on the hand and foot together, which may accelerate the body's response to the intention. It is a great technique in the toolkit of a reflexologist and can be used with the same method that I use in my therapy room – some palpations and sway, which help with rhythm and supports the delivery of my sessions.

Session 10, 15th December, 2021. Issues experienced by Fred, highlighted by parents, are at times discomfort with digestive difficulties and constipation. Of course, it is no surprise to reflexologists what the body can do for itself when we, as facilitators, encourage calm in the mind and the body may begin to relax. It may reduce discomfort, ease pain, ease digestive difficulties, reduce spasm and increase the feel-good factor.

Being an active listener when supporting a young person with profound and complex needs means listening and observing on many different levels.

Session 12, 12th January, 2022. My notes on this session remind me to remind you of the importance of listening, as following this session I wrote: 'Wow! Fred really made it clear today. [After] 12 minutes of calmness he removed his left foot first and slightly pulled back his right. I waited and then continued with some slow repetitive effleurage on his lower leg, he was quiet and "thoughtful" is a good word here, and for a second time he pulled back his feet.'

Interpret and respect

It is important, as I have mentioned previously, not to assume, but we do need to interpret and respect communication. I interpreted his movements and gestures, his stillness and quietness as his decision to end the touch session. I appreciated his communication, respected it, and concluded with the countdown.

I do regularly finish with close, quiet talking and sometimes the responses are beautiful. We can really have some fun together. What a great way for Fred to remember the reflexology sessions. I love the way our relationship developed.

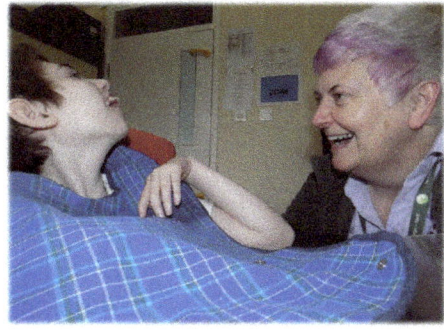 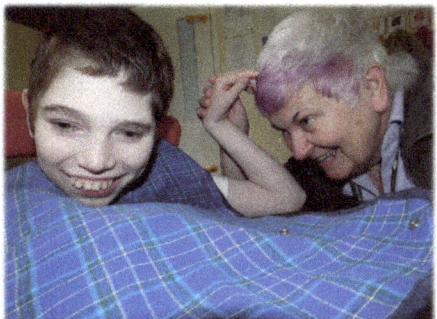

As we finish Fred is usually smiling and, if I am lucky, he will reach out and I receive a little hug. I'm sure it is his way of getting round me to stay in the therapy room for a few extra minutes. Cheeky! And yes, we do take a few extra minutes!

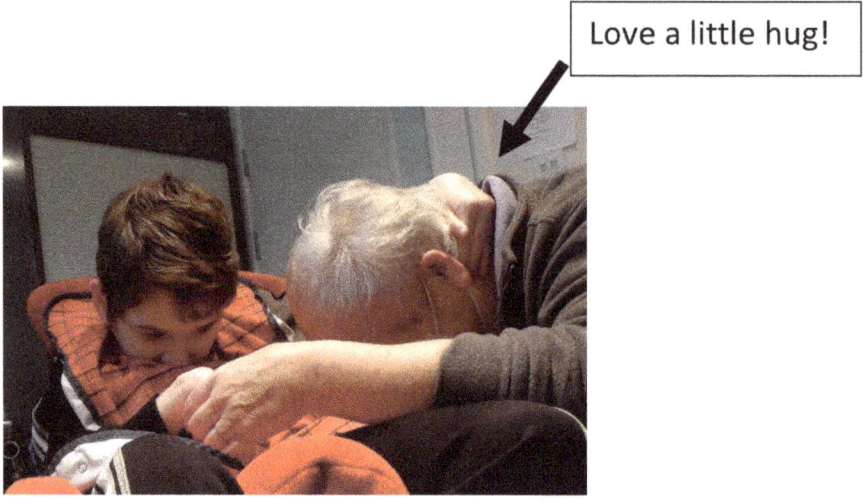

Love a little hug!

Efficacy and effectiveness

I have found that I use a variety of reflexology techniques to support Fred. My focus, with the repetition and rhythm of the delivery for relaxation, often centres on the digestive area, tailored to meet his needs.

He responds well through sound and body language to the slow effleurage up and down the lower leg (or forearm if I am working with his hands), the rhythm, the gentle swaying that I add in and the use of my voice. It is a combination that brings such value to the session and brings such a meaningful connection for supporting his well-being.

Teacher feedback

'I am aware that Fred can be frustrated, angry and quite distressed at times, and the reason I referred him is because I know how much he likes receiving nurturing touch and he does respond well to 1:1 attention and having time to make some choices. I was delighted to read the reports from Lorraine and to see some of the videos from the sessions. Fred recognises Lorraine's voice when she helps him prepare for the session, he certainly enjoys going out of the classroom as we get to hear wonderful noises as he disappears along the corridor. Time with Lorraine seems to help him to relax, and he returns generally happy.'

Feedback from Fred

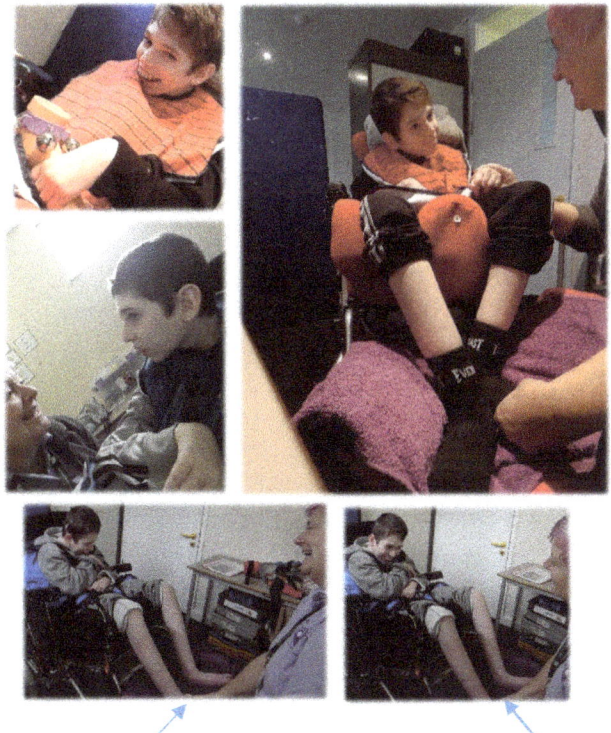

I wish the angle of the camera had shown my hold on his toes. But what it does show is his enjoyment of that sensation. Worth including!

Tips for Reflexologists

- » Use your skills and experience to provide the enjoyment of synergistic techniques, still delivered with repetitive movement, with palpation, and rhythm, and then the linking effleurage.
- » Using multisensory stimulation at transitions to help support an understanding and preparation of what is happening next.
- » Respectfully thanking the person who has come along to the therapy room. You may receive a surprising thank you back, but allow time.

Gratitude and Learning

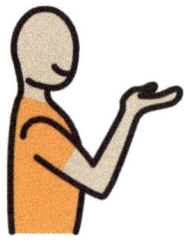

Thank You

Thank you, Fred, for accepting the invitation to come to the therapy room for reflexology. You have allowed me the opportunity to get to know you a little bit and not just to work with you. You have helped me to recognise the many benefits of working with a synergistic application of some techniques by listening and watching your responses. I loved your playful, 'cheeky' delaying tactics to extend time in the therapy room for extra time away from the busyness of the classroom! Thanks for the hugs!

Links and Further Information

Cerebral Palsy: www.cerebralpalsy.org.uk
PMLD Profound and Multiple Learning Difficulties charity: www.pmldlink.org.uk

Chapter 18: Meet Sharmin

'Sometimes I feel quite emotional at the end of my session with Lorraine, she says it's okay. Sometimes we sit still together, and she holds my hand.'

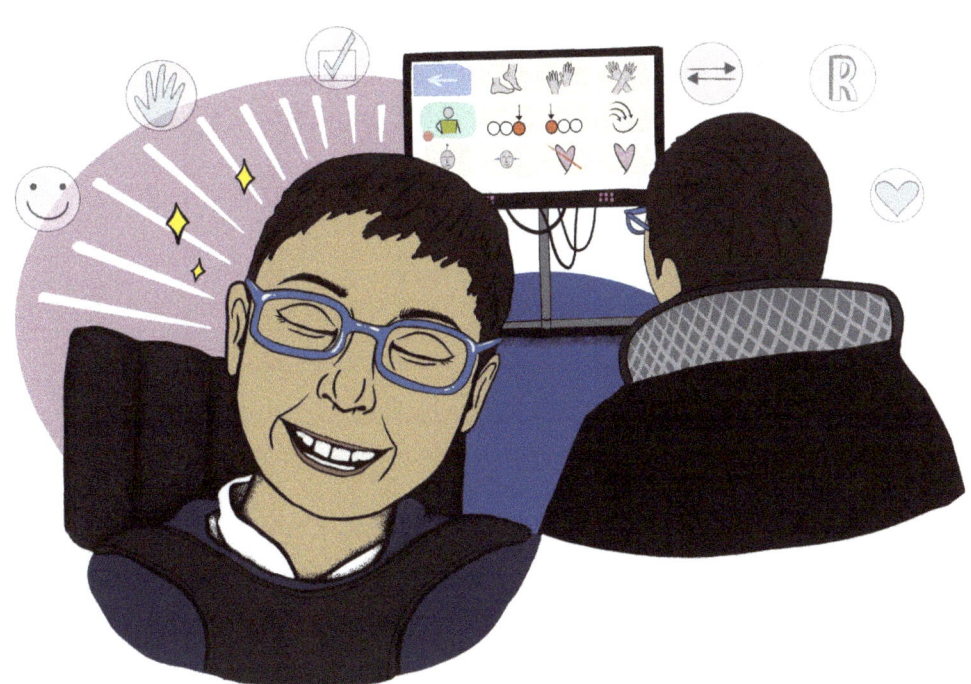

OUR WORK TOGETHER with individual reflexology sessions began in September 2021 when Sharmin was aged 14.

Sharmin and I were familiar with each other and we had developed a strong relationship. I had been supporting staff and young people in his class with the FRT Rainbow Relaxation activity for a number of years. He was familiar with my voice, with my touch, with the structured classroom activity, and I know he really enjoyed and benefited in a number of ways.

The FRT Rainbow activity has the same intention as my individual therapy sessions. The movements taught to staff are drawn from general reflexology and delivered with lots of repetition and rhythm to encourage relaxation through positive touch, but the individual reflexology therapy using the skilful techniques of the qualified reflexologist addresses much more.

Sharmin has bilateral spastic dystonic cerebral palsy, he has a learning impairment and quadriplegic CP and anisomyopia. These are conditions that can create discomfort throughout the body, which can cause worry, have an impact on emotional well-being, bring fretfulness, and raise anxiety levels.

The Process

Teacher referral

The teacher wrote, 'Sharmin loves to smile and warmly welcomes people who are familiar to him. He is a little more apprehensive when newly introduced. He does not use words but communicates through sounds, body movements and more recently in the last few years he has found his voice using eye gaze equipment, indicating preferences, making choices, and taking decisions using a choice of objects of reference or photographs.

'Sharmin can at times be sad, his mood may seem low, and he can seem very tired, which all affect how he manages during the school day.

'It is so important that we respect and encourage his engagement, make sure we allow sufficient time for him to make choices, and respect his decision.

'Poor sleep issues and sometimes discomfort with digestive problems can undoubtedly have an impact on engagement, learning and enjoyment of activities during the school day.'

The teacher wanted him to:

» experience 1:1 time away from the busyness of the classroom;
» have sufficient time to encourage communication, before, during, and after the session;
» be given some responsibility and the opportunity to make choices;
» have sufficient time and the opportunity to express his feelings;
» understand and feel in control of the activity;
» experience reflexology therapy to support well-being issues highlighted by parents (sleep and digestive);
» experience it to encourage raising his self-esteem and to let staff know how he is feeling when he returns to the classroom;
» generally, have fun through the sensory experience of reflexology, enjoying 1:1 attention.

Classroom observation

Although I had had the privilege of working with group sessions in the previous few years, it was important for me to undertake an observation session to focus on Sharmin. I dedicated the session to learning about how we could interact with eye gaze to give him some control and choices about reflexology. We would not have the option to use the eye gaze in the therapy room, but it would really support his communication before reflexology.

Using the eye gaze resources allowed Sharmin to make the decision about coming for reflexology. I would start with making sure that I was in view, and he knew I was talking to him: 'Good afternoon Sharmin'. I always showed the FRT toolkit and would place it on his tray or into his lap; sometimes I would also show a large photograph of Sharmin and me in the therapy room. He would often laugh and look to one side, perhaps bashful. Then, to allow time, I would remove the toolkit/photo so that he focused on the screen and was not distracted by squeezing the bag or giggling at the photo.

The question is, 'Would you like to go to the therapy room with Lorraine for reflexology?'

Sometimes, as you might have noticed from the eye gaze in the illustration, Sharmin might choose between feet and hands before we leave. I usually started with asking him if he wants to come and then, once in the therapy room, I can offer Sharmin a choice of hands or feet. As you will see in the gallery at the end of this chapter, he is good at positioning his head and eyes to let me know.

The reflexology session in the therapy room mirrors the beginning and end of the rainbow relaxation routine, and the delivery method, with flow, rhythm, and repetition aligns, but, as you will know, the techniques I use are often very different. They are tailored to meet Sharman's needs on the day.

Sometimes during the session Sharmin will make sounds that I interpret as what he uses to let me know he wants to tell me something. How do I know what he wants? Often, I don't! But what I do know is that I shouldn't assume I know: I need to allow him time and make methods of communication available that are appropriate for him.

Sharmin can make choices and can make decisions; he is able to shout out to let me know he wants to say something. (Not everybody is able to do this, and you will need different skills to identify and work with other people.)

The outcome may not always seem to be what you hope it will, but don't be fooled. Watch and listen. Only you can decide if there is a change for the better, no change at all, or a change that is not what you were hoping for or expecting. For example, you may feel sad if someone begins to get upset at the end of your session (or during it). After all, the intention of my sessions at school are to encourage someone to be calm, settled, and in a good frame of mind for coping with activities and enjoying learning. BUT … we can never truly say how the body may respond to the touch we are delivering or have just delivered, and releasing tension, time to think, reducing discomfort can all have an effect on your emotions. Being upset may not be such a bad thing, it might just seem so at the time.

Reflexology and reflection insights from my records

Session 7, 9th November, 2021. Sharmin and I would like to share with you a very personal example of the therapy experience. Please consider the value you can bring as a reflexologist 'beyond the touch'. When I collected Sharmin from the classroom I had noted a difference to his usual greeting. His head was lowered, he didn't deliver his usual smile and excitement. Staff commented that he had had a quiet morning and seemed a little tense.

As we began the session, I noted his arms were held in tight and his fingers quite curled and rigid. During the session he made a few unusual sounds that I didn't remember hearing before.

However, as the session neared its end, I felt his feet and legs gently relax and looking up I noticed that his arms had softened, his hands had lowered slightly, and his fingers seemed to have uncurled just a little. That brought me a little smile, as I thought I saw the benefits of my touch and the quietness of the environment in the way the body was relaxing.

While replacing socks and shoes, I was talking to Sharmin and telling him what I had noticed. I said, 'If you have been in some discomfort, or something has been worrying you, I am sorry I did not know. I hope you feel a little better now.' Over the next few minutes, as we sat quietly in reflection, he began to get upset and a real sadness surfaced. I'm getting emotional recounting that session as I write.

What did I do? I chose to hold his hand. He did not pull away, his hand rested on the back of mine as I placed it underneath and I placed my other hand on top. And we allowed a little time 'just being'. We sat together for a few minutes, and I generally talked about the session. I remember questioning myself: what was I talking about and was it meaningful, but, you know, sometimes just feeling a reassuring touch, hearing a calm familiar voice, gives meaning.

When I think back now as I type, none of us had many answers during the unsettled and disruptive years of 2020 and 2021. I found it very hard to make sense of, so what sense could Sharmin and many of the other young people I support make of it all? Could this be affecting how he was feeling? Or maybe it was nothing to do with that at all! I am just reassured that I had the reflexology environment to offer touch, kindness, and time to support as best I could 'in the moment'.

The sessions up to the Christmas break of 2021 were very quiet. Sharmin seemed a little subdued, but also there were many colds in school, along with illness caused by the Covid-19 virus. There were changes of staff in every classroom and some changes to the timetable were necessary. However, 2022 arrived.

Session 13, 11th January, 2022. Staff information on my arrival was that a change in the time of Sharmin's medication this week seemed to allow him to be much more engaged and alert. Maybe it was a combination of the Christmas break and the medication review? But it was great to see some smiles and hear some lovely sounds.

Choices and consent

Sharmin was using the eye gaze and particularly making his choice to go to the reflexology therapy room and for reflexology on his feet. Super choices and consent – thank you, Sharmin.

Teacher feedback

'When Lorraine enters the room Sharmin usually gets very excited. He lifts his head and waits with anticipation and a big smile for the preparation to begin.

'He enjoys her company and the 1:1 attention and I feel it is a valuable session for communication, relaxation, and emotional well-being.

'As Sharmin knew Lorraine well before starting the individual sessions, they had a good relationship already and the only new thing for Sharmin was going to a different part of the school visiting the therapy room. He usually arrives back content and we can see that he is quite relaxed. I feel it has more beneficial effects than just what we see on the surface on his return. How long his relaxed mood lasts may depend on what activity he is asked to do on his return!

'The sessions have been valuable, addressed many of the points on the referral sheet and Sharmin has really enjoyed the time with Lorraine.'

Efficacy and effectiveness

The most noticeable support that I feel came from the sessions was the focus on sufficient time. This is always so difficult in a busy classroom. Creating the right environment, allowing Sharmin the opportunity to be 'in the moment' and allow expression of feelings was so important for him. I was able to observe every movement and sound and to begin recognising preferred movements, which I could repeat.

Finishing reflexology completely can be difficult to understand for many of the young people who are invited to the therapy room. The preparation is just as important for finishing as it is for beginning the therapy sessions. I use a weekly countdown and verbal and visual information to try to provide meaningful information about stopping reflexology for that person. There is not enough time and space during the week to continue to see everyone, which is why the sessions are allocated with a finite number. Gosh, its hard though! I see the benefits for most young people receiving reflexology every week.

Think about positioning yourself and getting the young person's attention. Not necessarily insisting on them looking at you, but listening is crucial. Sharmin is really focused on the visual information, and I could tell he was listening to me. I am sure he understands.

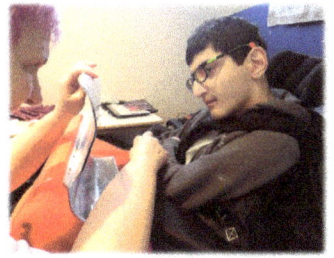 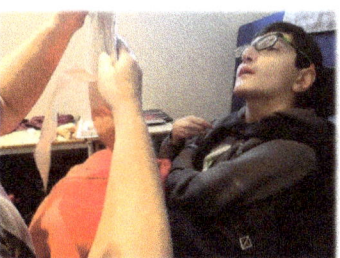 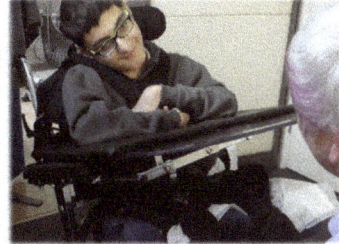

To complete our work together when we were back in the classroom, Sharmin was able to use his communication aid to say that he likes reflexology. I did ask if he understood that our sessions together had finished. The answer I got was a rather sneaky smile and side glance, as you can see. He wanted more.

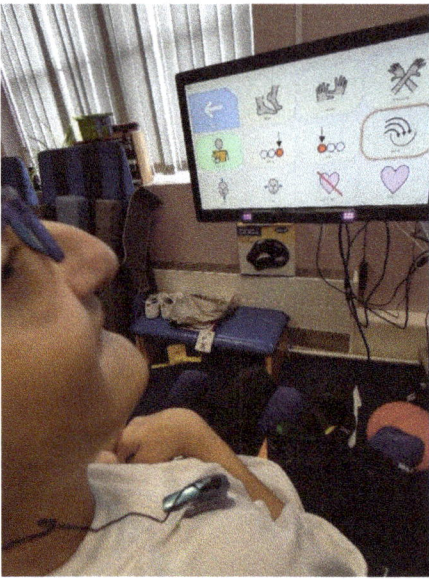

I absolutely love this ... the power of a photograph. What wonderful 'cheekiness' and such a fabulous respectful friendship had developed. Thank you, Sharmin. I hope you continue to enjoy the nurturing touch of reflexology in the future.

Just to let you know, over a year later Sharmin does still welcome me with a smile and beautiful sounds when I visit the classroom, so I feel we completed the sessions on friendly terms with a real value to our work together.

Feedback from Sharmin

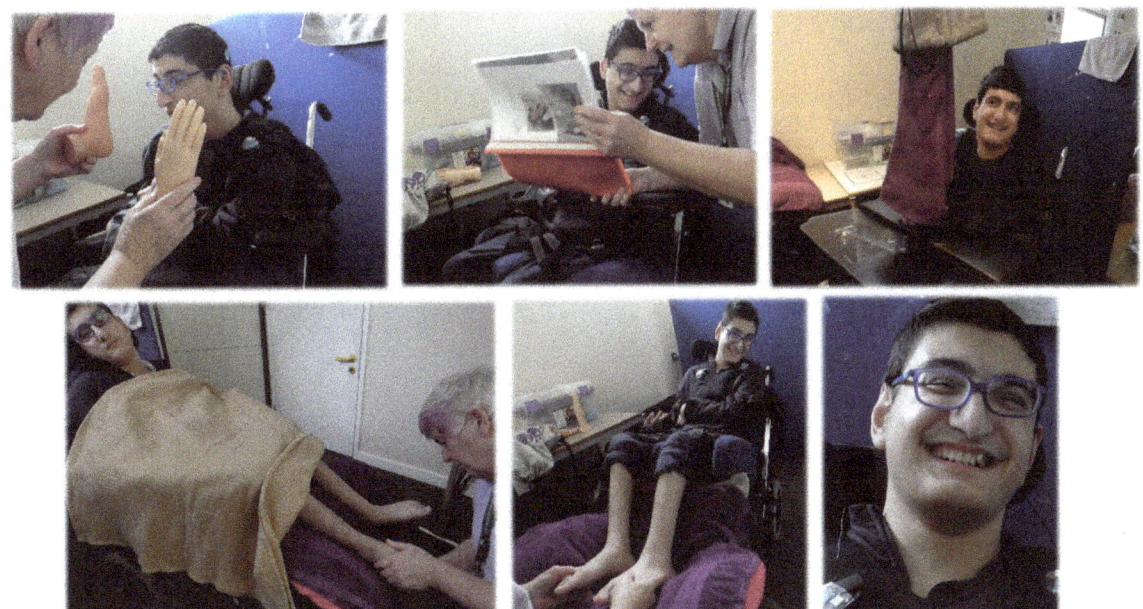

Tips for Reflexologists

» We can never truly say how the body may respond to reflexology, even in this short session with the intention for relaxation. Being upset could be the release that young person needed.
» To carefully listen should be part of your 'observation' – be an active listener.
» Remember the hands. You can offer great support for all areas just as you can the feet. For Sharmin, it was often a choice to complete the session with some time working on the hands.

Gratitude and Learning

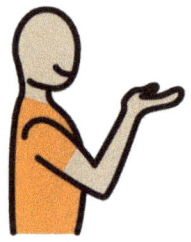

Thank you, Sharmin, for accepting the invitation to come to the therapy room for reflexology. You have allowed me the opportunity to get to know you and not just to work with you, which helped me to become a more respectful active listener. Thank you for your company, your genuine enjoyment of the therapy and for the fun and laughter we have shared.

Thank You

Links and Further Information

Communication Matters: www.communicationmatters.org.uk
Movement and coordination condition: www.cerebralpalsy.org.uk
Learning differences and intellectual disabilities: www.mencap.org.uk

Chapter 19: Meet Charlie

'I like the foot spa at the start and at the end I like the squeezing movement I do on my own hand.'

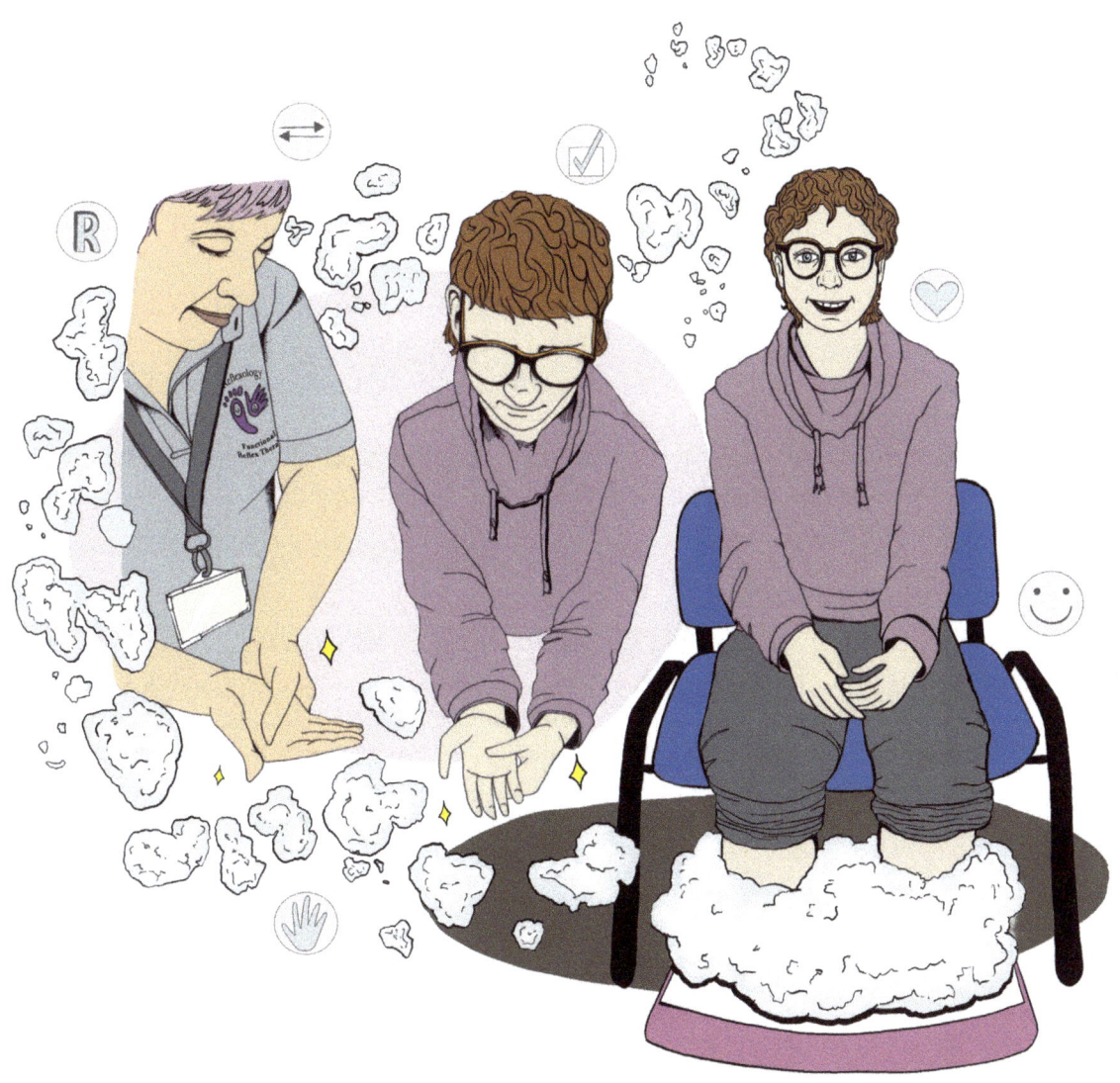

DURING OUR TIME in the therapy room throughout 2021 and 2022, we have enjoyed a lot of laughter together. I am delighted Charlie has chosen to write for you and that she is happy for me to share her work. Along with the teacher referral for the many benefits that you can bring through your reflexology and the general support of the session with the RECIPE of the Functional Reflex Therapy framework, please enjoy Charlie's story.

The Process

Teacher referral

'Charlie is generally a happy young lady at school. She has some language and learning difficulties which have affected her confidence and sometimes finds it challenging to acquire and maintain some key skills. She does bring her worries to school; it can often show itself with her feeling angry, being anxious or quite the opposite, being very quiet and at times seeming withdrawn within the classroom.

'Due to Charlie's quietness and shyness, I wanted a supportive therapy that was quiet, reflective, and tailored to suit her personality; self-care was key, as with her anxieties, she was struggling with coping and being kind to herself.'

The teacher would like her to:

- » have fun and relax with a short time away from the busyness of the classroom to participate in something just to focus on herself and raise awareness of self-care and well-being;
- » be encouraged to lift self-esteem through the session;
- » use the reflexology therapy room as an environment where she feels relaxed and has an opportunity to express her feelings, perhaps her thoughts and any worries;
- » be provided with the opportunity to make choices and decisions within the therapy room, which may build confidence;
- » consider that, if this is an experience that she enjoys, perhaps she will have an opportunity to consider reflexology as part of her lifestyle in the future.

Classroom observation

It was helpful for me to spend time in the classroom. Charlie was very quiet. I noticed her watching her friends, but often she lowered her gaze to avoid them if they looked at her.

Many of her answers to questions were given with a nervous giggle, a raise of her shoulders, and an 'Urm, I dunno,' – good, or not sure?

Reflexology and reflection insights from my records

It was always important to welcome Charlie with a reassuring greeting, calm voice, and positive comments. I always found something good to comment on; it truly sets the scene! How do you greet your clients? Think about the intention and purpose of your session beyond the touch of your reflexology. Charlie did not physically need the FRT toolkit, but your welcoming tool, your approach, your voice, your reassurance, is part of your toolkit.

It was important for me to reassure Charlie each week and let her know this was her time, she can talk about anything, or she can enjoy the quietness, which is what she did most of the time. I do recognise when she is beginning to relax, and on just a few occasions, with my encouragement, she closed her eyes.

A Few Words Shared from Charlie

Hi, my name is Charlie, and I am 19 years old, my birthday is in October.

I like coming to school. I walk to school. I really like English and Drama.

I am quiet.

I have lots of friends.

I asked Charlie if she feels anxious about anything or worries about things.

Sometimes I worry about doing new things. Meeting new people.

I love cooking. I like baking. I bake a lot at home and my favourite cake to make is chocolate cake.

I go for reflexology with Lorraine every Tuesday at 9.15

In the therapy I take of my shoes and socks and I use a foot spa to clean my feet. Sometimes I turn the bubbles on and they go over the top, we laugh a lot together how far will I let the bubbles grow. Lorraine says I always have lots of fluff from my socks.

I sit in the big chair it goes back and I have cream on my feet. Lorraine always asks me if I would like a blanket, I always say no.

Lorraine does movements on my feet, and my on my legs.

I like it. It makes me happy, and I smile. Sometimes I close my eyes it feels different when I close my eyes, but I don't know why.

> The best thing I like is time out of class. I like all the movements, but I like it on my toes the most.

> Lorraine asks if I would like to come back next week.

We have been discussing what the movements feel like on Charlie's feet if anywhere feels uncomfortable and what that feels like. I am encouraging her to describe how they feel and trying to raise awareness of any internal feelings. eg warmth, cold, tingly, this is very difficult.

Here I am in the big chair enjoying reflexology.

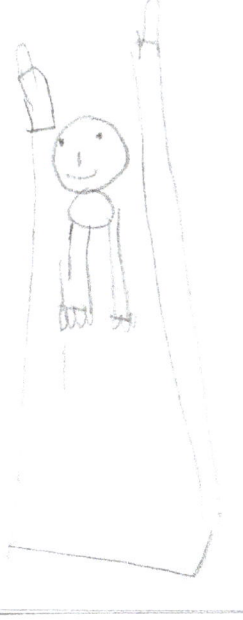

Efficacy and effectiveness

Very early on, I brought self-care into the session, introducing the foot spa. It was a great decision! It really helped bring some fun and chat into the therapy room. There was also an important intention, too, that we could talk about foot health, nail care, and hygiene.

As the weeks have progressed Charlie seemed a lot more comfortable with my company, she has settled into the routine of the sessions and is interacting with a lot more confidence. For example, a few sessions ago (session 14), I said, 'Goodness, I see lots of fluff in the foot spa today – have you got new socks?' 'I think it must be your eyes' was the reply, with lots of laughter. I know this may seem a slightly odd comment for me to pop into a reflexology report, but, as you already know, the therapy sessions in school are so much more than 'just the touch of reflexology'. Wow … we laughed and it highlighted a little cheekiness but mainly how much more relaxed and comfortable Charlie was feeling.

By session 8, I had added empowerment and responsibility into our time in the therapy room. I said that I would continue to deliver reflexology until Charlie said she was ready to finish, so I put her in charge of bringing the session to an end. I wanted her to be in control and to voice that. It made Charlie smile when I said that it might be a problem if she didn't tell me to stop and we had to keep going all morning! (Yes, I did have a cut-off time to bring the session to a close if she hadn't asked me to finish.) But, fortunately, it worked well.

Teacher feedback

'Charlie has always been shy and demure, however I noticed that the anxiety was more than introversion. After setting up a plan with Charlie to support her through this time she was finding challenging she was willing to take time away from the class just for her. She was already familiar with Lorraine the reflexologist having joined in some class self-care sessions.

'On returning to the classroom after attending the reflexology sessions, the classroom staff began to notice a difference in Charlie. Within four sessions she seemed more alert and a little more willing to contribute. She started to eat and drink healthier foods and started to take a little pride in her appearance.

'With every "touch" of positive energy from the therapy room the best way I can describe her transformation was that she blossomed and started to talk about issues. She started to resolve problems and talk a little more to her friends. She became a cheeky and happier student. Her mindset was focused, and she excelled in her exams attaining a higher level than predicted at the start of key stage 5.

'The original plan for reflexology was to meet the criteria already mentioned. However, for Charlie the whole framework along with the enjoyment of receiving the touch lowered her stress and has given her a much improved quality of life.

'On returning from the sessions, she spent a better quality of learning time with teachers which in turn saw her progress as mentioned with her higher-level achievement. It gave her the confidence to talk to her peers and she has realised she could create boundaries, make decisions, and say no.

'She seemed generally less overwhelmed and is coping well. She really enjoyed the sessions; she has dealt better receiving praise and positive touch. She has even shared her reflexology experience with her peers.' (A T, 2021)

Feedback from Charlie

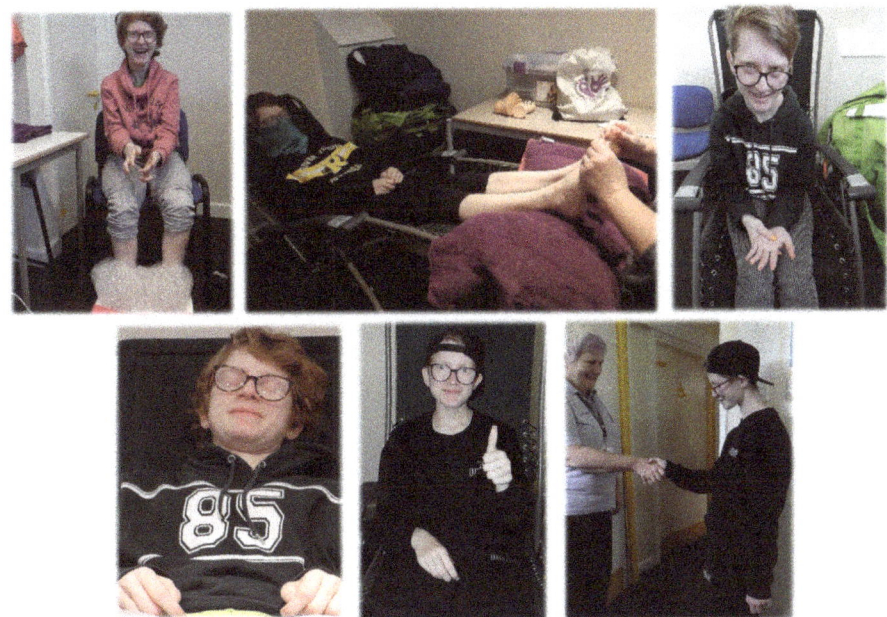

Tips for Reflexologists

» Be aware that different sensations may be felt with delivering to both feet at the same time, as opposed to one foot and then the other. Offer a choice, allow your young client to feel both, and work with their preference.
» Teach self-care techniques for the hands and arms, skills that are transferable and can be used in and outside of school.
» Never underestimate the power of your therapeutic relationship, and what you can help to develop through your respect, fun, and kindness of the nurturing touch of reflexology.

Gratitude and Learning

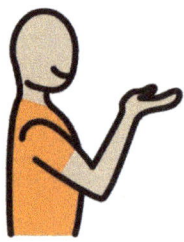

Thank You

Thank you, Charlie, for accepting the invitation to come for reflexology. Our sessions were so much more than the touch of reflexology. We have managed lots of laughter, especially with a lot of bubbles in the foot spa. One of the nicest parts of work together was when you were able to describe a little visualisation. Well done learning the self-care activities, I hope you find them helpful and you enjoy their continued use.

Note: Reflexologists and headteachers, enjoy this story, but please make sure you read and re-read the teacher feedback.

Chapter 20: When Headteachers and Reflexologists Meet

School: Harlow Fields School and College
Headteacher: Kathleen Wall
Reflexologist: Lorraine Senior

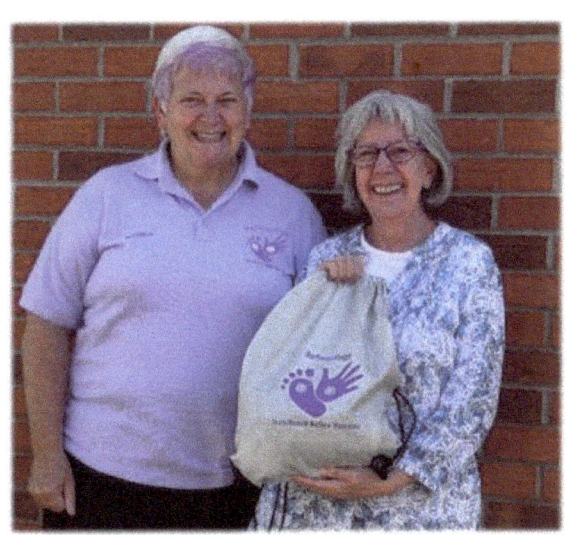

Headteacher's contribution (submitted 2017)

Many of our young people, especially those who have autism, like to be, or feel they need to be, in control of every minute of their life. Reflexology gives them time out of class, allowing somebody else to be in control, helping them to give up or reduce their control, to relax and enjoy a positive form of touch.

The students are very aware that when they see Lorraine, something lovely is going to happen. They recognise the logos that she has developed, it helps with meaningful communication and recognising what is going to be offered and will happen.

She has developed a toolkit for her reflexology which encourages our young people to get involved in the sessions. Many of them like the bag and like to see what is inside. They recognise her trademark colour purple and that they are either going to have a session in the classroom or special 1:1 reflexology time with her. The logo and bag help them prepare for that.

Many pupils use the 'first and then' strategy and the logo or Lorraine's photo is used to help them to understand what is happening.

We know the children enjoy the session by the fact that they just love going with Lorraine. Importantly, they show us by the way they are much calmer in class afterwards, and by the way they become much more willing to enter the therapy room area. If it is a new area, sometimes they are quite reluctant at first, then gradually, over a period of time, they become more comfortable with the session and the touch and may even choose the relaxation touch activity in the classroom, so they show us in lots of different ways that they enjoy it.

Lorraine is just part of our team now; I couldn't imagine life at Harlow Fields without her. She has shown us a whole different therapy, a whole different way of interacting with the children. We've always had a therapy based curriculum for some of our children and therapeutic interventions, but not all children respond to a talking therapist or music therapy, for example. The young people needed something different and Lorraine has brought a whole new way of interacting with our children and we have seen such benefits in terms of their learning and relaxation. Lorraine contributes to all our reports and will run workshops to support our parents, which is very useful for them, and she is just part of our team.

Lorraine's contribution (reflexologist)

During my time at Harlow Fields School and College I created workshops and have been sharing the FRT Rainbow Relaxation Routine with parents and with staff for them to use in the classroom. It is similar, yet different, to my work delivering reflexology.

This is an additional pathway for FRT. Delivering workshops for parents and carers is available to all reflexologists that hold current membership of the FRT Network. And some FRT reflexologists are now developing their business to offer workshops for school staff.

I asked my headteacher this very important question: 'Does my sharing do me out of a job?' and received a very reassuring answer:

'No! Certainly not! Because we know that the two are different. The rainbow therapy can be delivered by a whole range of people, and I think for our young people this is important for the touch to continue two or three or more times per week if possible or on a regular basis. It does not take away from the 1:1 touch that you provide as a reflexologist. Different things, yet they complement each other with the similar structure and start and finish and it's all about receiving nurturing touch, but you are not doing yourself out of a job.'

School: Hayfield School, based in Merseyside, UK
Headteacher: Mr L. Comber, Deputy Head: Ms S Wilson
Reflexologist: Debbie Hurst

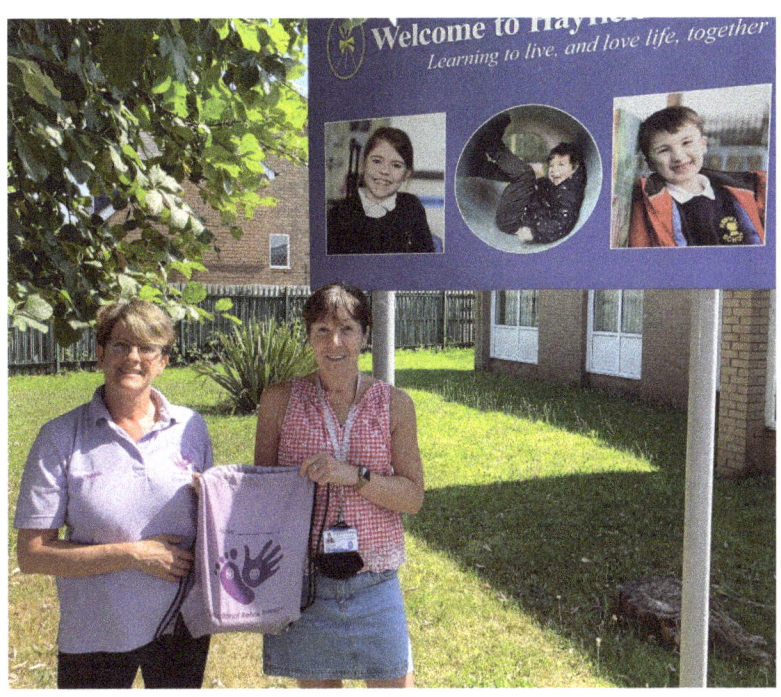

Contribution from Sue Wilson (Deputy Head)

(submitted 2021)

Hayfield School is a specialist primary provision for children with additional needs. The majority of children have a diagnosis of autistic spectrum condition. However, the school supports children with a range of difficulties, including social, emotional, and mental health issues, children with attachment trauma and children with moderate and complex learning needs.

We have been fortunate to have a trained reflexology practitioner (Debbie Hurst) working with cohorts of our children for a number of years.

As part of our multi-disciplinary approach, staff identify children who it is felt will benefit from sessions of reflexology supported by the FRT framework. There is a substantial amount of preparatory work that takes place before the child has their first session. Staff work with Debbie to identify particular and individual needs of the child, and the session is tailored and adapted to meet these needs. As a practitioner in a school, Debbie has to be flexible, adaptable, and creative when delivering her reflexology sessions and the FRT framework helps support this. Debbie works with the children in a session of between 15 and 20 minutes. Within that time Debbie will be cognisant of the individual child's needs; this might be to support sensory difficulties, hyper or hypo arousal, support anxiety, prepare the child in terms of supporting attention, and so on. Ultimately the experience is for the child. Many of our children thoroughly enjoy the sessions and are very motivated. A considerable number of children that Debbie works with have considerable anxiety (for a variety of reasons).

It is very clear that the delivery of the reflexology sessions and her approach has a significant impact on their ability to be able to 'switch down' that anxiety. Our children can find it difficult to label their emotions and the therapy has enabled some of them to at least be able to feel the big differences in the feeling of anxiety to that of the feeling of calm when they are in a session. There were also effects on the children's toileting habits. A lot of the children can suffer with constipation and often reflexology sessions would help relieve their stomach pain.

The children benefit enormously, and often that benefit spills over into a following lesson (or even for a good part of the day) where the child is notably calmer, more relaxed, and much more able to focus.

Overall, we are very fortunate to have Debbie working at Hayfield School. Reflexology has such a positive impact on our children in so many ways. They thoroughly enjoy the sessions (from their feedback). Debbie has an excellent understanding of the children's needs, and both the parents and school are very grateful for the benefits provided by regular/timetabled reflexology sessions.

Reflexologist's contribution

I feel very fortunate to be working at Hayfield School, delivering reflexology supported by the FRT framework as part of a child's weekly timetable.

The teachers identify children they believe would benefit the most from this therapy, which helps to calm and balance their nervous system. It is usually children with high anxiety levels, and/or difficulties concentrating in class. I treat six children in a morning, which is generally about half a class, but split over different classrooms.

I love watching their faces as they relax in the chair, close their eyes and, with the slow breathing, start to really unwind. Sometimes it is just a short 5, 10, or 15 minute session that really helps them take 'time out' to switch off and connect with how they are feeling. Equally, I love the 'thumbs up' and smiley faces I get at the end.

I have had fantastic feedback from both parents and teaching staff. One mum's feedback: 'Yes she was much calmer than usual on Friday evening, she also puts her feet up on my lap for a foot rub so she must be enjoying the sessions!'

Feedback from staff: 'I have seen a vast improvement in pupils' behaviour, being able to regulate behaviour and feelings/emotions, being able to access class activities after attending a session of reflexology.'

I passionately believe that these reflexology treatments make a difference. The children genuinely look forward to them.

Reflexology at Transition2 in Derby
Janine Cherrington (Head of Service)
Seema Ghai (Reflexologist, Foot Care Specialist)

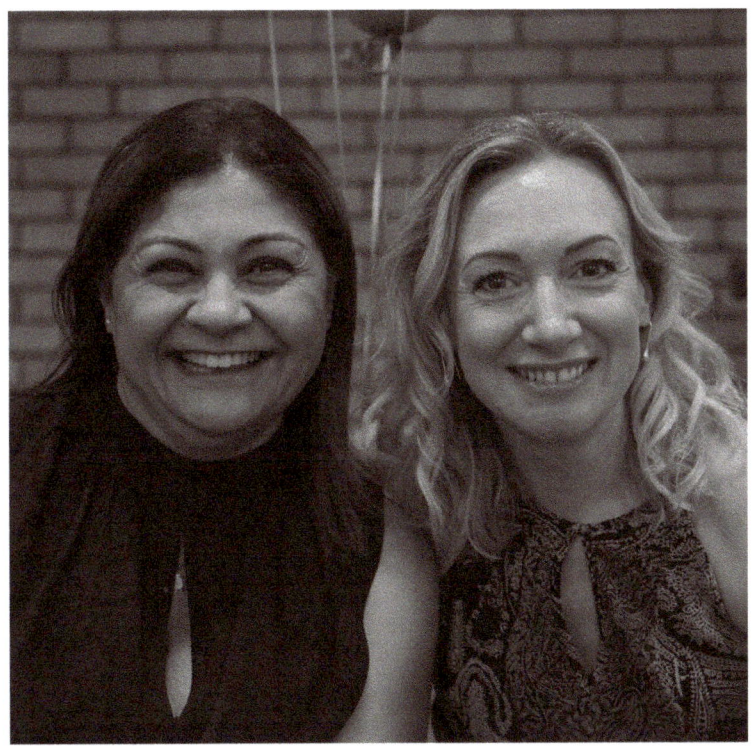

Janine Cherrington's contribution (submitted 2021)

Transition2 has embedded somatic practices into our learning offer since we opened in 2012, including reflexology supported with FRT with our qualified reflexologist, Seema. Through our work in The Thrive Approach, we recognise that a well-functioning autonomic nervous system is a key foundation for cognitive processing and learning outcomes in all young people, especially learners such as ours, who have severe learning disabilities, global developmental delay, autism, mental health challenges, or complex needs.

Listening to the feedback from our bodies through interoception is crucial for the development of neuroceptive skills in self-regulation, which underpins learning potential in the neo-cortex; the strategies employed with the delivery of FRT therefore act as a catalyst for the development of self-management skills and independent thinking.

Using the unique method of FRT to deliver reflexology helps learners to connect with their breath, heart rate, temperature, bodily sensations, and emotions in a way that is calming and intimate but non-threatening, through the offer of dedicated time, quiet attention, and positive, safe touch. For learners who may experience volcanic eruptions in emotion, anxiety, or behaviour, reflexology sessions supported with the FRT method are a special time when they can experience deep feelings of safety; as a result, they may choose to share personal stories or memories, or explore some of their barriers to learning. The calming effect of the sessions also offer the opportunity for learners to practise essential independence skills, such as removing their own shoes and socks or waiting patiently outside the therapy room for their appointment.

When you see the impact that reflexology supported with the FRT framework can have on emotional regulation, cognitive processing and memory recall in learners who have received it, you'll agree that every school needs a Seema!

Reflexologist's contribution

My name is Seema Ghai, and I am a qualified reflexologist and use the FRT framework to support my sessions at Transition2 (also known as T2), based in Derby, Derbyshire. T2 is an education facility for young adults aged between 18 and 25 with severe learning difficulties, learning disabilities and/or autism.

Learners are usually referred to me as part of their curriculum, or because they have complex issues, and I usually see 3–4 learners per session.

I have been delivering my reflexology sessions at T2 for the past seven years and it has provided me with a simple sequence to use on learners that they can become familiar with very quickly! Over the years, I have had the privilege to offer FRT workshops for parents and carers so they can use the Rainbow Relaxation Routine at home to promote relaxation and well-being.

I highly recommend the FRT course with Lorraine for reflexologists and the FRT Rainbow Relaxation workshops for parents and carers, which may be offered by a qualified therapist in your local area.

Youthreach, Kilkenny, Ireland
Michelle Murphy, Co-ordinator/Comhordaitheoir
Reflexologist: Geraldine Duffy (Submitted 2021)

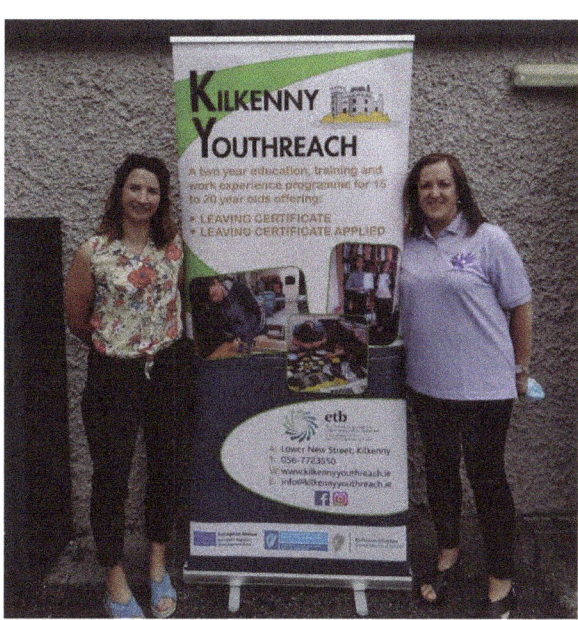

Michelle Murphy's contribution (submitted 2021)

Youthreach is a high support setting, and having a professional reflexologist delivering reflexology supported by the FRT framework on site once a week is a fantastic addition to the range of supports we provide. It became an important dimension to our support system and one that our students eagerly await each week.

Our reflexologist had a weekly slot and quickly became an important part of the wider programme here. The students enjoyed the regularity of this slot and are comforted by the sense of routine it instilled. Prior to commencing any treatments, the reflexologist addressed each class and explained exactly what they could expect from the session. She also gave a demonstration; this eased any unknown anxiety the students may have had.

For us, reflexology delivered and supported using the unique approach of FRT provided a space of calm for students that needed it. This calm certainly had a lasting effect and teachers regularly commented on the positive change in a student's demeanour after their reflexology session.

We intend to continue providing the reflexology framework to our students once a week. Our reflexologist is in tune with the needs of our students, and they reap the rewards of this contact at each visit. It is a fantastic addition to any school's support system.

Reflexologist's contribution

I commenced reflexology, which I support using the FRT method of delivery, in this second level school with three students. Many knew nothing about reflexology, some had heard the word, so it was a good time to raise awareness of the principles of reflexology and how it can support young people during the school day.

The students I support were able to tell me they feel very relaxed following the session, and they all mentioned that they felt it helped them to sleep better.

When they present, sometimes it is evident that moods may be very low, and this may be for many different reasons. The intention of the reflexology session is to help them to be in a better frame of mind, which may help them to cope better during the school day. I try to create a safe and calming environment; they may feel they can talk, or they may just close their eyes and relax. Each person reacts differently. The important question I ask myself is: 'Do they leave the therapy room in a better frame of mind?'

I use the FRT structure within the session, but I do not need to use the FRT toolkit with the students I currently support.

The structure, timing, purpose, and intention of the session makes it ideal for the timetable during the school day. Students are referred if they have difficulties coping and may have high levels of anxiety.

Being in this privileged position as a reflexologist using the FRT Framework to support the well-being of young people during the school day, when they may be finding it difficult to cope, gives me such a buzz. It is wonderful to see its many benefits of support and the students are so open and receptive.

I would love to see more secondary schools open their doors and welcome qualified reflexologists using the FRT framework to see its many benefits and value for their young people and the staff.

School: Endeavour Academy
County School Based in Oxfordshire
Headteacher: Michaela Soporova
Reflexologist: Anne Spencer

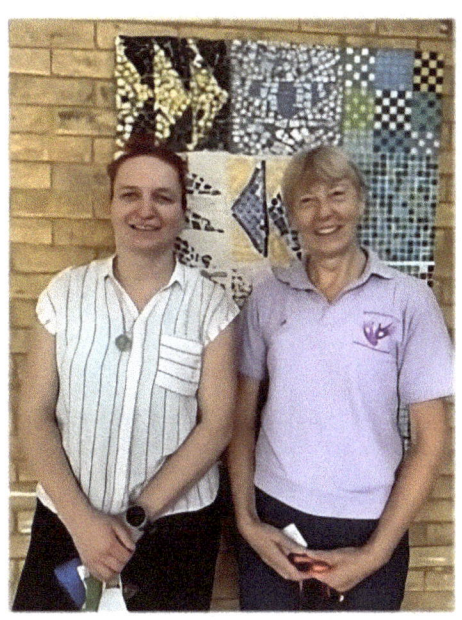

Headteacher's contribution (submitted 2021)

Anne, a qualified reflexologist, has been supporting students at Endeavour Academy for a number of years. Our students have autism and severe or moderate learning disabilities and many also have additional sensory difficulties as well as anxiety and health complications. Most are not able to fully explain their problems and needs. Since working with Anne, who introduced the reflexology therapy and the support of FRT with its framework and many supportive pathways, we have recorded decreased levels of anxiety in a number of our students. Her knowledge and skills support our multi-professional discussions, and she has provided training to further support our staff, who are now able to deliver aspects of FRT in the classroom through the Rainbow Relaxation Routine, which supports the role of the reflexologist.

We have a number of students who were initially hesitant about attending reflexology with Anne who are now not only fully engaged, but actively seeking Anne when she is on their timetable.

Reflexologist's contribution

I have supported the Endeavour Academy using the FRT framework alongside the delivery of my reflexology since October 2016. I currently attend two days a week, working with up to 12 pupils.

Most of the pupils I support are non-verbal and have significant behavioural challenges. The pupils I work with are nominated by the class teachers, who select those they deem most in need of/most likely to benefit from the sessions. It takes some pupils a while to understand the 'process', that is, coming from the classroom, sitting in the reflexology chair and receiving the therapy, but they soon look forward to it, choose whether they want the chair reclined or upright, blanket or no blanket, and relax well. It is important to provide meaningful communication and sometimes the FRT toolkit can really help with their awareness and preparation.

As I am delivering the session, I observe how they are on arrival, how they relax during the session, the level of interaction in the form of eye contact/smiles, whether any elements of the sequence cause them to wriggle or feel uncomfortable (commonly the digestive system!). It is a valuable way to interpret and understand issues a pupil might have, especially as they are not able to verbalise or communicate where they might be in pain or uncomfortable.

It is so lovely and such a privilege to be recognised and respected as a valuable member of the multidisciplinary team, to be able to offer a few minutes' quiet away from the classroom, some individual time and space to relax, to help them to be in a better frame of mind to cope as best possible as they return to the classroom.

Rowan Park Special School (Complex Needs & Autism, 3-19 years)
Rowan High (Autism Pupils Aged 11-19)
Location: Sefton, Merseyside.
Reflexologist: Janet Hardman (Contribution Submitted 2021)

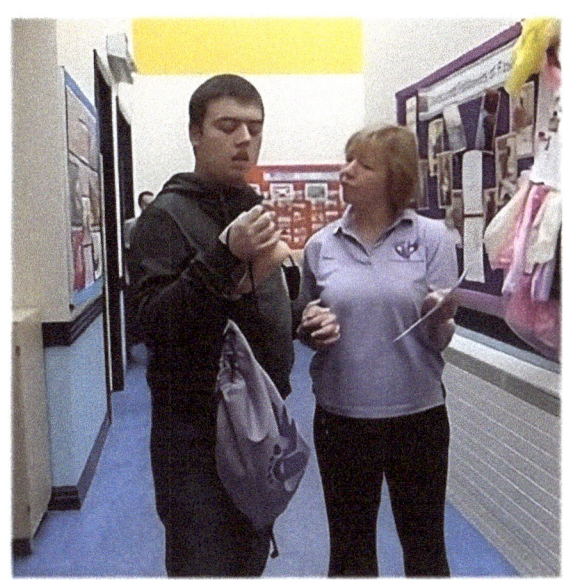

I started delivering reflexology therapy supported with the FRT framework in 2014. The course material provided by Lorraine during the training provided me with very helpful information which I used to support my presentation to the school governors, highlighting its many benefits and value of a therapy to have on the timetable.

As a special school teacher, specialised in developing communication, and a reflexologist, I was very aware of the benefits of, and need for, therapeutic approaches to be part of the curriculum.

Most importantly, the FRT framework supports the schools' approach to developing 'Total Communication', that is, the teaching of a variety of different communication strategies – signing, use of objects of reference, photos, symbols, and symbol timetables.

The FRT framework has an additional benefit to 'our' pupils as it offers a simple routine that can be shared with parents and carers through a workshop, empowering parents with additional skills, benefiting both parents and pupils. I have guided many parents through the workshops, and they have generated a lot of interest. Schools are always looking to provide courses for parents, too.

When a teacher refers a pupil, before sessions start, I discuss with the teacher and class staff the pupil's Individual Education Plan (IEP) and targets, so that, as well as my session target of encouraging relaxation in that moment, I can address their targets that are set in class from B. Squared (a method of assessment demonstrating small steps of progress and achievement). Very quickly the staff recognised that they and the pupils were benefiting from the sessions.

Chapter 21: Final Words

MY INTENTION BEHIND this book was to share the power of reflexology and to encourage reflexologists to consider developing their business with the FRT framework. I want to offer a structure and consistency, supportive documentation, delivered with purposeful intent. There is immense value in supporting the emotional well-being of young people during the school day.

I hope that you have seen how you can apply these tools to support young people who are managing a range of challenging difficulties, symptoms of anxiety, and complex conditions and diverse needs. I have used many labels and names, and while these conditions cannot be cured, they do not disappear, nor are they grown out of. Reflexology therapy is a supportive intervention and strategy. When we can offer it to young people, we can provide an opportunity for them to better manage, regulate, and thrive during their school years and beyond, so they feel good about themselves and boost their self-esteem.

It is truly a privileged position to know that you could make just a little difference 'in the moment' of a young person's day. Outside of the classroom and outside of the school day can trigger many anxieties, too, and FRT reflexologists can support with many pathways.

As reflexology therapists, we often work in isolation in our therapy rooms or clinics and talk only with our clients (and ourselves), but being part of the multidisciplinary team brings a connection on so many levels and allows you to truly begin to understand the young person you are supporting.

When I look back, not just at the stories within my book, but on almost every referral form I have received throughout the years in school, the words most often mentioned are communication and time, which I have mentioned throughout the book. Time away from the busyness of the classroom and time to allow information to be gathered, processed, and responded to. This has to say something about our education system. Of course, sufficient time is only valuable if you have the right methods of supportive communication in place to allow each person to tell you how they are feeling or share their worries and, importantly, have an opportunity to exercise a choice.

If the most ticked box is time away from the busyness and noise in the classroom, perhaps we need to look at how we can create a more appropriate environment. The invitation to receive reflexology would, of course, still be very valuable for well-being but it wouldn't be used as much as needed at present for escaping the busyness, and when the young person returns to the classroom they may continue their learning in a more 'friendly' environment.

If I had not spent time in the classroom, if I had not had times when I found it challenging to reach out and try my best to communicate with some of the young people, if I had not taken time to consider and question what I could have done differently, how I could deliver a different approach, I would not have written this book. And if I had assumed and presumed I knew best, I most definitely would not have written this book. If I had not listened to, and learned from, the young people in the classroom who showed me the advantages and benefits of nurturing touch, I would not have followed the pathway seeking the many benefits of positive touch in schools.

If I had not spent years struggling with a physical hindrance through early onset osteoarthritis from the age of 40, I probably would not have taken steps to begin my training in reflexology.

Sometimes, in our world today, things are wanted and expected 'just like that'. We seem to have forgotten, or are too quick to dismiss, what can happen by allowing time for ideas to develop and for ongoing learning.

Allowing ourselves time, giving ourselves permission to take time to grow our minds and experiences, is vitally important, as is time to consider how we might best use these experiences for the benefit of others. Giving time to our approach, allowing time in the delivery of our reflexology, as we communicate through our touch, for the body to make sense of the information we provide and time to respond to it.

My years of regular support in school have offered consistency to many pupils and a very different experience for them. With this has come the privilege to get to know each person in a friendly space and not just work with them.

I hope that working in school and doing what I have been talking about for so many years, developing the framework as my work progressed, will be helpful and give confidence to reflexologists to realise that there is real value in taking your therapy into school. I hope, too, that it will impart confidence to headteachers that there is real value in welcoming a qualified reflexologist, using this focused professional package and framework, as a valued member of their team.

A qualified reflexologist with, often, many additional areas of expertise, but importantly supported with the FRT framework and its many pathways and a consistent intention for it to be available during the school day and in every school throughout the world, can introduce a well-being experience for young people, for schools, for staff, and for parents.

Reflexologists, I know the school environment is not for everyone. We all have our interest and our passions. Schools deserve to have reflexologists that are passionate to become members of the team. You need commitment and to provide and develop your skills perhaps in a different direction to your current one, but it is such a valuable pathway and reflexologists deserve to have schools that are looking for and respect a qualified reflexologist and the value they can bring in as part of the team.

Parting Gift

I received this lovely gift at the end of a presentation day with the British Reflexology Association. Sally wrote it during the final session and shared it with us all at the end of the day. I wish I could capture the lovely rhythm she used as she read to the group, her beautiful tone, and the thoughtfulness of her voice. Perhaps you will find it yourselves in the lines and words.

I continue to remain very touched that my day spent with you inspired these words with realisation of its many pathways of support. *Thank you.*

Take a moment to enjoy Sally's words.

Functional Reflex Therapy
For emotional health
Can support a parent
To empower themself

Providing nurturing touch
To reduce anxiety
Enables their loved ones
To find harmony

Communication is the key
With special needs
Repetition and Rhythm
Process then succeeds

The vision to deliver
Reflexology
To all schools and care homes
Supporting FRT.

Sally Price 2018
Member of the British Reflexology Association BRA
Senior Lecturer in Health & Wellbeing, University of Wolverhampton

Where Do I Go from Here?

There are many pathways within FRT through which the reflexologist can offer valuable support.

- » Individual reflexology therapy with the support of the FRT framework involves the reflexologist 'blending their ingredients' through the FRT RECIPE, carefully considering their approach before, during, and after reflexology. Importantly, I ask them to consider reducing the number of changes of reflexology techniques with attention to the glabrous and non-glabrous skin areas. The method of delivery offers repetition and maintains a reassuring rhythm to allow the body time to get familiar with the movements and time to receive and process the information communicated through touch.
- » FRT Rainbow Relaxation workshops, on the other hand, are offered by FRT reflexologists to support parents, carers, and family members with skills to use in the comfort of their own home at a time that is right for them. Together these platforms can foster good home–school links.

If you are a reflexologist and have found the Functional Reflex Therapy framework and stories inspiring, and you would like to know more about its many pathways and how to develop your business to introduce your work to schools and to support families, you can find out more at www.functionalreflextherapy.co.uk

If you have picked this up as a teacher or headteacher because you've been directed to the book or because you are interested in finding out how to support your young people further, this could be the beginning of reflexology supported by the FRT framework on the timetable in your school and the opportunity for you to welcome a qualified FRT reflexologist as a member of your multidisciplinary team.

You can find out more at www.functionalreflextherapy.co.uk

About the Author

Lorraine Senior, B.Ed (Hons)

Founder of Functional Reflex Therapy (FRT), Lorraine is a qualified teacher, with over 20 years of experience working within the mainstream and special education system, and over 14 years as a qualified reflexologist.

Combining her teaching and reflexology experience, working with both children and adults with additional, complex, and diverse needs, Lorraine has adapted and combined techniques through the approach of the FRT RECIPE and the supportive FRT toolkit. She has raised awareness of the importance of allowing time, providing meaningful communication, and the value that increased repetition of reflexology techniques and the rhythm of the delivery can provide for reducing anxiety and supporting emotional well-being in readiness for learning during the school day.

Now she is sharing her work to encourage reflexologists to introduce the value of reflexology supported by the FRT framework into a variety of environments, including schools. Lorraine feels very privileged to provide support and ongoing training for qualified reflexologists and, since the courses were introduced in 2014, has worked with over 500 therapists who are now using the approach to support their business. The training for reflexologists is currently three days face to face and, following the course, reflexologists have ongoing support through access to an active network of FRT reflexologists and a members' area.

Lorraine continues to deliver in-house training in schools and to professionals seeking to introduce the FRT Rainbow Relaxation programme into their professional environment.

She provides informative, fun, practical workshops for the family to prepare them to use the rainbow relaxation routine in the comfort of their own homes.

In 2017, Lorraine created the FRT Global Projects. It continues to develop as the FRT team works alongside education colleagues in both the Southern Province and Lusaka Province in Zambia, Africa to train teachers and young people in the many benefits that the kindness of the nurturing touch of reflexology, through a structured activity, can bring to help calm and focus the mind within the classroom.

Lorraine is the proud recipient of three wonderful awards:

- 2016 the Winner of the Association of Reflexologists Award for Excellence and Innovation in Reflexology.
- 2017 the Winner of the Federation of Holistic Therapists Tutor of the Year.
- 2019 A Humanitarian Award from the International Council of Reflexologists for the supportive work of the FRT Global Project Zambia.

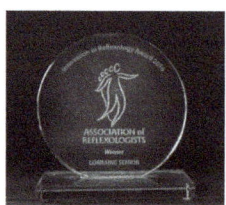 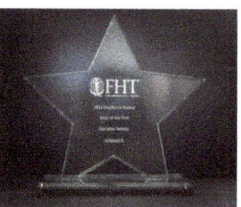 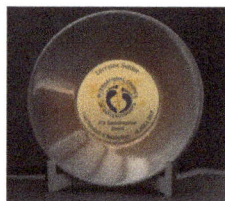

You can find out more about the many benefits and the many pathways that are available at www.functionalreflextherapy.co.uk

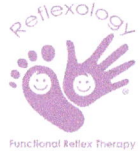 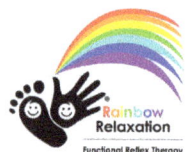 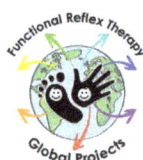

Useful Resources

1p36 deletion syndrome www.rarechromo.org
ADHD Neurodiversity Charity www.adhdfoundation.org.uk
Association of Reflexologists www.aor.org.uk
Augmentative and Alternate Communication AAC www.slt.co.uk
Blepharitis www.nhs.uk/conditions/blepharitis
Cardiofaciocutaneous Syndrome www.cfcsyndrome.org
Cerebral Palsy www.cerebralpalsy.org.uk
Communication Matters www.communicationmatters.org.uk
Down's Syndrome Association www.downs-syndrome.org.uk
Epilepsy Society www.epilepsysociety.org.uk
Hypothyroidism www.nhs.uk/conditions/underactive-thyroid-hypothyroidism
Juvenile Arthritis www.arthritis.org/diseases/juvenile-arthritis
Lafuma Chair www.lafuma-furniture.co.uk
Learning Disability www.mencap.org.uk/learning-disability-explained/what-learning-disability
Makaton Language Programme www.makaton.org.uk
Mencap www.mencap.org.uk
Mental Capacity Act 2005 (MCA) NHS Health Research Authority British Institute of Learning Disabilities www.bild.org.uk
National Autistic Society www.autism.org.uk
Objects of Reference and Communication www.sense.org.uk
Profound and Multiple Learning Difficulties www.pmldlink.org
Reflexology supported with the FRT Framework during the School Day https://www.youtube.com/watch?v=xWOaO7Bfq6c
Schwachman-Diamond Syndrome www.sdsuk.org
Sensory Processing Difficulties www.sensoryspectacle.co.uk
Social Stories www.carolgraysocialstories.com
Speech and Language Therapy www.rcslt.org/speech-and-language-therapy
Verrucas and Warts www.nhs/conditions/warts-and-verrucas
Weighted Blanket www.sleepfoundation.org

Bibliography

Akarsu, R., Öztürk, B., & Karatekin, C. (2020). Investigation of the effect of sensory integration therapy and foot reflexology applications on sensory modulation and sleep in a case with autism. *International Journal of Basic and Clinical Studies*, 9(2): 114–121.

Atkinson, M. (2009). *Healing Touch for Children*. London: Gaia Books.

Beardon, L. (2020). *Avoiding Anxiety in Autistic Children: A Guide for Autistic Wellbeing*. London: Sheldon Press.

Bidwell, V. (2016). *The Parents' Guide to Specific Learning Difficulties*. London: Jessica Kingsley.

Bjornsdotter, M., Ilanit, G., Pelphrey, K. A., Olausson, H., & Kaiser, M. D. (2014). Development of brain mechanisms for processing affective touch. *Frontiers in Behavioural Neuroscience*, 8(24). Available at: https://www.ncbi.nlm.nih.gov/pmc/articles/PMC3912430/

Booth, L. (2000). *Vertical Reflexology*. London: Judy Piatkus.

Brown, B. (2021). *Atlas of the Heart*. New York: Random House.

Cullen-Powell, L. A. J., Barlow H., & Cushway, D. (2005). Exploring a massage intervention for parents and their children with autism. The implications for bonding and attachment. *Journal of Child Healthcare*, 9: 245–255.

Dorman, P., Aldridge, J., & Fraser, B. (2006). Using students' assessment of classroom environment to develop a typology of secondary school classrooms. *International Education Journal*, 7: 906–915.

Edgar, H. (2016). *Limbic Reflexology: Student Textbook*. Self-published.

Escalona, A., Field, T., Singer-Strunck, R., Cullen, C., & Hartshorn, K. (2001). Brief report: Improvements in the behavior of children with autism following massage therapy. *Journal of Autism and Developmental Disorders*, 31(5): 513–516.

Field, T. (2000). *Touch Therapy*. London: Churchill Livingstone.

Field, T., Lasko, D., Mundy, P., Henteleff, T., Kabat, S., Talpins, S., & Dowling, M. (1997) Autistic children's attentiveness and responsivity improve after touch therapy. *Journal of Autism and Developmental Disorders*, 27(3): 333–338.

Gale, E. (2002). Advocating the use of reflexology for people with a learning disability. In P. A. Mackereth & D. Tiran (eds), *Clinical Reflexology: A Guide for Health Professionals* (pp. 159–169). London: Churchill Livingstone.

Grace, J. (2022). Share their picture, say their name. Is it safe to share photos of people with profound intellectual and multiple disabilities online? The ethics of being presented to the online world. *PMLD Link*, *23*(2): 103.

Higashida, N. (2021). *The Reason I Jump: One Boy's Voice from the Silence of Autism*. London: Sceptre Books.

Hirstwood, R. & Gray, M. (1995). *A Practical Guide to the Use of Multi Sensory Rooms*. UK: Toys for the Handicapped.

Hudson, D. (2015). *Specific Learning Difficulties: What Teachers Need to Know*. London: Jessica Kingsley.

Ishak, W. W., Kahloon, M., & Fakhry, H. (2011). Oxytocin role in enhancing well-being: A literature review. *Journal of Affective Disorders*, *130*(1–2): 1–9.

Kedar, I. (2012). *Ido in Autismland*. Sharon Kedar.

Kranowitz, C. S. (2022). *The Out-of-Sync Child. Recognising and Coping with Sensory Processing Disorder* (3rd edn). New York: TarcherPerigee.

Kunz, K. & Kunz, B. (1996). *Reflexology for Children*. Scotts Valley, CA: CreateSpace.

Lavrinĉik, J. & Tománková, K. (2020). Research of hand reflexology stimulation in children with ADHD. *Cognitive-Social and Behavioural Sciences*, vol. 1. *European Proceedings of Educational Sciences* (pp. 143–152). https://doi.org/10.15405/epes.20121.17

Li, Q., Becker, B., Vernicke, J. et al. (2019). Foot massage evokes oxytocin release and activation or orbitofrontal cortex and superior temporal sulcus. *Psychoneuroendocrinology*, *101*: 193–203.

Longhorn, F. (1988). *A Sensory Curriculum for Very Special People*. London: Souvenir Press.

Mackereth, P. & Tiran, D. (eds) (2002). *Clinical Reflexology: A Guide for Health Professionals*. London: Churchill Livingstone.

Osgood, T. (2019). *Supporting Positive Behaviour in Intellectual Disabilities and Autism: Practical Strategies for Addressing Challenging Behaviour*. London: Jessica Kingsley.

Panksepp, J. (1993). Commentary on the possible role of oxytocin in autism. *Journal of Autism and Developmental Disorders*, *23*(3): 567–569.

Pistorius, M. (2011). *Ghost Boy*. London: Simon & Schuster.

Porges, S. W. (1991) Vagal tone: a mediator of effect. In: J. A. Garber & K. A. Dodge (eds), *The Development of Affect Regulation and Dysregulation* (pp. 111–128). New York: Cambridge University Press.

Reardon, T. C., Gray, K. M., & Melvin, G. A. (2015). Anxiety disorders in children and adolescents with intellectual disability: Prevalence and assessment. *Research in Developmental Disabilities*, *36*, 175–190.

Riquelme, I., Hatem, S. M., & Montoya, P. (2016). Abnormal pressure pain, touch sensitivity, proprioception, and manual dexterity in children with autism spectrum disorders. *Neural Plasticity*, *2016*, doi: 10.1007/s10803-011-1214-0.

Spratt, E. G., Nicholas, J. S., Brady, K. T., Carpenter, L. A., Hatcher, C. R., Meekins, K. A. et al. (2012). Enhanced cortisol response to stress in children in autism. *Journal of Autism and Developmental Disorders*, *42*(1): 75–81.

Uvnas-Moberg, K. (2003). *The Oxytocin Factor*. Stockholm: Natur Och Kultur.

Uvnas-Moberg, K., Handlin, L., & Petersson, M. (2015). Self-soothing behaviours with particular reference to oxytocin release induced by non-noxious sensory stimulation. *Frontiers in Psychology*, *5*. Available at: https://pubmed.ncbi.nlm.nih.gov/25628581/

Voos, A. C., Pelphrey, K. A., & Kaiser, M. D. (2013). Autistic traits are associated with diminished neural response to affective touch. *Social Cognitive and Affective Neuroscience*, *8*(4): 378–386.

White, S. W., Oswald, D. Ollendick, T., & Scahill, L. (2009). Anxiety in children and adolescents with autism spectrum disorders. *Clinical Psychology Review*, *29*(3): 216–229.